Thrive Through Menopause

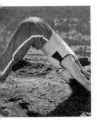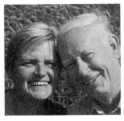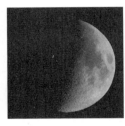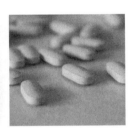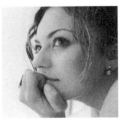

52 Brilliant Ideas

one good idea can change your life

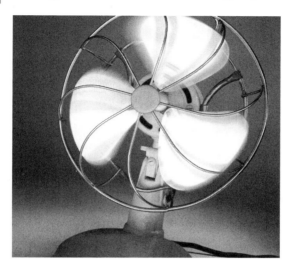

Thrive Through Menopause

Smart Ways to Feel Great and Enjoy the Prime of Your Life

Monica Troughton

A Perigee Book

A PERIGEE BOOK
Published by the Penguin Group
Penguin Group (USA) Inc.
375 Hudson Street, New York, New York 10014, USA
Penguin Group (Canada), 90 Eglinton Avenue East, Suite 700, Toronto, Ontario M4P 2Y3, Canada
(a division of Pearson Penguin Canada Inc.)
Penguin Books Ltd., 80 Strand, London WC2R 0RL, England
Penguin Group Ireland, 25 St. Stephen's Green, Dublin 2, Ireland (a division of Penguin Books Ltd.)
Penguin Group (Australia), 250 Camberwell Road, Camberwell, Victoria 3124, Australia
(a division of Pearson Australia Group Pty. Ltd.)
Penguin Books India Pvt. Ltd., 11 Community Centre, Panchsheel Park, New Delhi—110 017, India
Penguin Group (NZ), 67 Apollo Drive, Rosedale, North Shore 0632, New Zealand
(a division of Pearson New Zealand Ltd.)
Penguin Books (South Africa) (Pty.) Ltd., 24 Sturdee Avenue, Rosebank, Johannesburg 2196,
South Africa

Penguin Books Ltd., Registered Offices: 80 Strand, London WC2R 0RL, England

While the author has made every effort to provide accurate telephone numbers and Internet addresses at the time of publication, neither the publisher nor the author assumes any responsibility for errors, or for changes that occur after publication. Further, the publisher does not have any control over and does not assume any responsibility for author or third-party websites or their content.

THRIVE THROUGH MENOPAUSE

Copyright © 2007 by The Infinite Ideas Company Limited
Cover art by SuperStock
Cover design by Liz Sheehan
Text design by Baseline Arts Ltd., Oxford

First American edition: August 2008
Originally published as *Magical Menopause* in Great Britain in 2007 by The Infinite Ideas Company Limited.

Perigee trade paperback ISBN: 978-0-399-53437-9

PRINTED IN THE UNITED STATES OF AMERICA

10   9   8   7   6   5   4   3   2   1

PUBLISHER'S NOTE: Neither the publisher nor the author is engaged in rendering professional advice or services to the individual reader. The ideas, procedures, and suggestions contained in this book are not intended as a substitute for consulting with your physician. All matters regarding your health require medical supervision. Neither the author nor the publisher shall be liable or responsible for any loss or damage allegedly arising from any information or suggestion in this book.

Most Perigee books are available at special quantity discounts for bulk purchases for sales promotions, premiums, fund-raising, or educational use. Special books, or book excerpts, can also be created to fit specific needs. For details, write: Special Markets, Penguin Group (USA) Inc., 375 Hudson Street, New York, New York 10014.

Brilliant ideas

Brilliant features

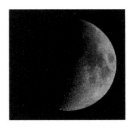

Each chapter of this book is designed to provide you with an inspirational idea that you can read quickly and put into practice right away.

Throughout you'll find four features that will help you get straight to the heart of the idea:

- *Here's an idea for you* Take it to heart and give it a try—right here, right now. Get an idea of how well you're doing so far.

- *Try another idea* If this idea looks like a life-changer then there's no time to lose. *Try another idea* will point you straight to a related tip to enhance and expand on the first.

- *Defining idea* Words of wisdom from masters and mistresses of the art, plus some interesting hangers-on.

- *How did it go?* If at first you do succeed, try to hide your amazement. If, on the other hand, you don't, then this is where you'll find a Q and A that highlights common problems and how to get over them.

Introduction

It is a magical time—honestly. This is said straight from the heart of a woman in her early fifties who is right there with you now as you go through menopause.

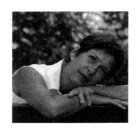

No one looks forward to menopause, partly because of all the bad press it receives and partly because menopause is about the end of a time in your life linked to fertility, and that alone can make you panic. As if that isn't enough, you read that you are now becoming one of the elite "hags" or "crones." Those words still suggest "witch" to me. Who on earth wants to be called a "crone," a "hag," or even a "wise woman"? I don't! I felt those terms were alien and excluded me from everyone around me. This was the last thing I wanted—especially when I was feeling a little odd anyway. I was also fed up with pointing out to people that not too long ago women really were the wise ones—they held the keys to power, dished out the herbs, and healed people. I hoped that if I said positive things about women and their menopausal years I might feel a bit better about having started mine. But it didn't work, and I still felt old and dreaded anyone knowing. I had a real fear that my femininity had been taken away from me and was a little bit scared I'd look like one of those toothless hags I had seen in fairy-tale books as a kid.

On the other hand, if you associate menopause with trips to your doctor and medical center then the chances are that you might view menopause as an illness, which it clearly isn't. Even though you might feel as though you are going around the bend at times, menopause still isn't a sickness. I wanted ways to get through it without being dependent on drugs or medical intervention. I don't particularly enjoy being told what to do, and a lifetime ahead marked by wearing a hormone patch (which I tried) as a constant reminder that I was no longer "normal," or popping a pill I didn't really want to take, didn't feel right for me. But I did want something to help me through.

I started to explore the options I had. What could I take to make sure my skin stayed in tip-top condition? What was happening to my body? Would my sex life dwindle to nothing? I wanted to know so much and by talking to women who were going through it, and by consulting dozens of experts, I found out that there is a lot you can (and have to) do for yourself.

You might find that some of your symptoms are too hot to handle and that you need and appreciate some support from your doctor or nurse. That's fair enough. You have to do what you think is right and proper for you. By choosing your own support mechanism you are liberating yourself and becoming a very strong woman. You don't have to follow any set of hard and fast rules for menopause. Through using this book as a guide you should be able to discover ways to work with menopause so that you get the most out of it. After all, what's the point of going through all those changes if there's nothing to be gained from them? You don't even have to wait until it's over to reap the rewards of menopause; they are with you every day. The more you help yourself, the more you stay in tune with your body, your mind, and your soul. The more you track your own symptoms and respond to them in a positive way, balancing your mind and body, the more liberated and powerful you become. As soon as you become the mistress of your own well-being you feel better. As soon as you take responsibility for your menopause you will find every area of your life improves, from your physical to your emotional and spiritual health.

This book is crammed with everything you need to know about how to stay strong and healthy from day one of your menopause right to the very end. I promise you that when you read it and realize the full potency of menopause, you'll only want the best for yourself and nothing short of that will do. You might find you become a little bit scary, too—well, good. There's no harm in being a little fearsome now and then, especially if you have always been afraid to say *no* in the past. In fact, as you make progress through your menopause you will discover and enjoy new and important aspects of yourself that you had no idea were even there.

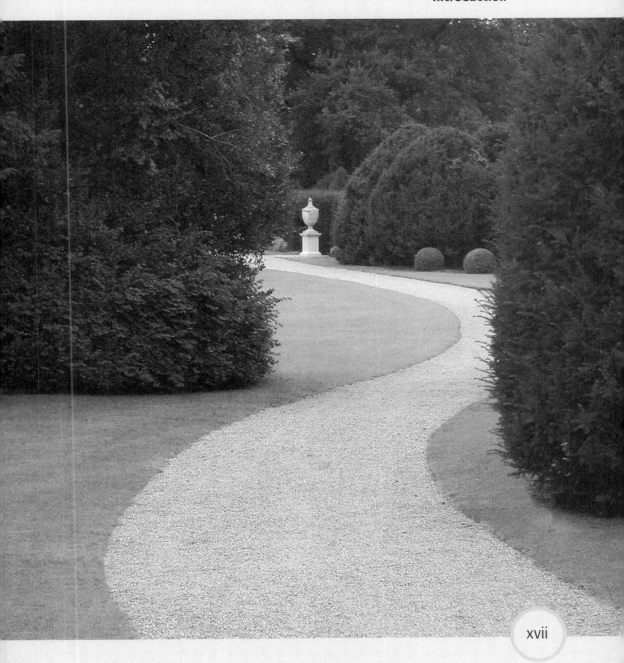

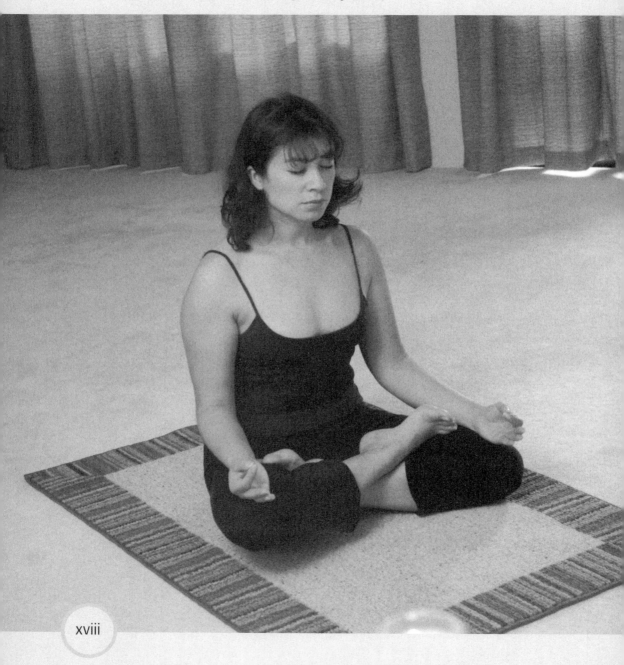

1

Bent double

Yoga is great for a healthy menopause.

You might not have considered yoga
before and although it isn't an overnight
fix, you will respond very well to it.

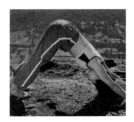

Yoga has so much to offer and it works on so many levels—meaning you can't help but enjoy menopause once you work with it this way. Some of the best (and best known) poses are Child, Hare, Little Bird, Dynamic Breath, Cobra/Sphinx, Bow, Fish, and Camel.

Yoga stretches can benefit both your body and your mind, bringing energy and balance. This is particularly good for you if you are feeling out of balance with your fluctuating hormones at the moment. Yoga exercises level out this instability by relaxing and gently stretching every muscle in the body, promoting better blood circulation and oxygenation to all cells and tissues. In turn this will help your endocrine system function better. This is good news during menopause because this system is responsible for secreting hormones directly into your bloodstream from various glands such as the thyroid, pituitary, ovaries, pineal, and adrenals. Yoga exercises also improve the health and well-being of your digestive tract and nervous system, and all your other organ systems.

Many yoga exercises address specific menopause-related symptoms and issues, such as the strength of your bones, cardiovascular system, and breast health. Yoga can also help alleviate menopausal symptoms such as insomnia, depression, hot flashes, and mood swings. The deep breathing and relaxation prescribed by yoga is beneficial in improving blood circulation, maintaining muscle tone and flexibility, and increasing the levels of mood-regulating chemicals in the brain, among other things. Yoga actually massages the internal organs, nourishing them with increased blood circulation, as well as toning the interior and exterior muscles. I think that's pretty impressive, don't you?

Here's an idea for you…

If there isn't a yoga class where you live then why not buy some yoga videos and practice poses in the privacy of your own home? You could get a few menopausal friends together and have a yoga night. Many yoga videos or DVDs cover the whole ability range from beginners to the more advanced, so you can be sure of finding something that suits you.

Not only is it working wonders for you during menopause but your body will look pretty good after a course of yoga—and the beauty is that you can practice it at home away from class, so the benefits will be with you every day.

When doing yoga exercises, it is important that you focus and concentrate on the positions. First, let your mind visualize how the exercise should look, then follow with the correct body placement for the pose. The exercises are done through slow, controlled stretching movements. This slowness allows you to have greater control over your body movements. You minimize the possibility of injury and maximize the benefit to the particular area of the body where your attention is being focused. Pay close attention to the initial instructions.

The following pose might be part of a complete yoga routine that can help alleviate menopausal symptoms. It is one you could practice first thing every morning and last thing at night to help remove any tension in your body. It emphasizes good posture and breathing.

- Stand up straight with your feet together. Extend your arms straight up toward the ceiling.
- Inhale deeply.
- As you exhale, slowly bend forward, letting your arms move down but keeping them straight, and allow your head to hang down gently. Try not to bend your knees.
- Inhale and slowly come back up to a standing position.
- Repeat twice.

The idea is to relax. So, don't force your body; never cause pain. The biggest mistake beginners make is to overindulge. These are not quick-fix solutions; natural remedies work

Try another idea...

While yoga is helping restore and rebalance you, you might want to focus on IDEA 30, *Gasping for air*, for how to breathe properly and make the most of oxygen as you practice your yoga poses.

Defining idea...

"The yoga mat is a good place to turn when talk therapy and antidepressants aren't enough."
AMY WEINTRAUB, author and founder of Life Force Yoga Healing Institute

gently with the body over time. As you reap the rewards, though, you will have a clearer understanding of how your body is working, especially through menopause. Why not make yoga part of your daily routine from now on?

How did it go?

Q Since menopause I have been suffering from painful joints and they have definitely tightened up so I am nowhere near as supple as I used to be. Is yoga a good idea for me or might it make my condition worse?

A   *Yoga is most definitely right for you. Over time you will notice an improvement in your mobility and you should become more supple. You will probably notice the pain in your joints is also relieved as your overall system becomes toned.*

Q I'd love to do yoga but suffer from the most awful flatulence brought on by menopause. I'm terrified I'll embarrass myself in the middle of a tricky pose and don't attend a class because of this. How can I prevent this from happening?

A   *The yoga teacher I asked about this told me that she always warns her students not to worry about flatulence because some of the poses she teaches actually help relieve trapped wind: She thought it was a positive thing. If you are really windy these days, maybe you should examine your diet and see what's creating the excess flatulence. Avoid this particular food on the days you have yoga.*

2

Warming up for the real thing

The part before the real thing is known as "perimenopause" and lets you know menopause is on its way.

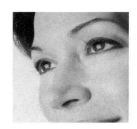

If you are in the perimenopausal stage then you could feel some of the symptoms normally associated with menopause, but in a diluted way— and you're still having periods.

Some physicians say perimenopause can last between five and fifteen years, while others argue that it's the four to five years before your final period, and includes the first year after that. So there's no clear view on how long it takes or exactly when it happens, except that the general agreement is that it takes place somewhere between the ages of 35 and 50!

The symptoms of perimenopause are what most physicians do agree on, and these symptoms are very similar to those of menopause itself. Perimenopause means that

Here's an idea for you...

Note the trigger for your hot flashes. Sugar? Caffeine? Alcohol? Spicy food? As soon as you see a pattern developing you will know what to cut down on or eliminate from your diet. Although hot flashes might happen with alarming frequency, as often as every few minutes, they actually only last for a matter of seconds and are not constant. You could go for months without a single flash even after you've had a couple. Wear loose, comfy clothes you can whip off discreetly if you need to. Tight and restrictive clothes could make you feel as though you are going to explode, and so are best left in the closet for the time being.

your hormonal system is beginning to prepare you for menopause, and in doing so begins to throw up all sorts of menopause-like symptoms. But not everyone experiences it. Just as you might have suffered from period pains when you started puberty while your best friend didn't, so it's the same with perimenopause.

Look for the following:

- occasional hot flashes
- mood swings
- insomnia
- irritability
- vaginal dryness
- forgetfulness or lack of concentration
- changes to your periods in that they might become heavier, lighter, or more irregular

It's unlikely anything will happen that you can't or won't be able to deal with in a positive way.

Unlike menopause, your perimenopausal symptoms won't be constant. The general rule of thumb is that when your periods cease altogether you'll know you are fully menopausal. You might find this stage a bit daunting and confusing as the symptoms might vary and won't be consistent, but your body is making adjustments and knows what it's doing.

Being prepared and ready to make some last-ing changes in your life at this stage should make the transition to menopause less of a challenge and possibly more interesting. It will definitely contribute to how you experi-ence menopause and could even make it easier to go through.

There are herbal remedies you can take to help you on your way. Black cohosh is avail-able in pill form or as a tea. It has remarkable properties (and can even be used as an antidote should you ever be bitten by a rattlesnake). More conventionally, it's alleged to alleviate hot flashes and depres-sion, and it can really help you if your energy seems to have left you. Black cohosh is somewhat of a wonder herb and it is claimed that it can ward off headaches, reduce high blood pressure, and be really very useful if you are considering alternatives to conventional HRT. Other herbs you could check out are phytoestrogen-rich dong quai and red clover, as both are known to help with perimenopausal symptoms.

Your health will benefit at this time if you can reduce your caffeine intake and drink herbal teas instead. Try supplementing your diet with:

- Vitamin E, to improve vaginal dryness
- Magnesium, to keep osteoporosis at bay
- Omega-3 and omega-6 fatty acids, to improve calcium absorption and bone density

Growing older is as natural as every other cycle you've been through. But if perimenopause leaves you mourning your loss of youthfulness and in a sweat about aging, then see IDEA 5, *Hanging on to your bits and pieces*, for ways to keep everything in shape.

Try another idea…

"Yes, I'm 53 years old, but I don't think about it. I only think of what I must do tomorrow—that I must dance Swan Lake, that I must dance Sleeping Beauty."
MARGOT FONTEYN

Defining idea…

Once you have put a program or regime into place to help ease symptoms, you can rest assured your body will get on with it and leave you to carry on with your life. Overall, like any transition, your perimenopause is exciting because it heralds the dawn of a new era—and nothing will be the same again. As with everything new, it takes time to become familiar with the changes but once you have done so you will experience a calmer and wiser attitude toward your menopause.

How did it go?

Q How will I definitely know I am going through perimenopause?

A *If you have any symptoms associated with your menstrual cycle or hormonal changes then you could see your doctor, who will arrange a blood test to check hormone levels. You can also buy hormone testing kits from pharmacies and health stores, which will give you a good idea about your hormone levels. They work in the same way that pregnancy tests work.*

Q OK, I think I am perimenopausal—I am more tearful now—but I am still having regular periods. Is this normal?

A *Perimenopausal women often have regular periods so you have to look out for other symptoms. Perimenopause can often strike just as women are at the peak of a career or suffering with a relationship issue. Your hormones aren't behaving in a predictable manner and this can create havoc with your emotions. If you monitor, listen, and deal with the demands your body is making right now, then perimenopause will be a lot less stressful and will actually make you a stronger woman, more than able to deal with issues that need tackling head-on.*

3

Use those green fingers

You may silently snicker "Yeah, right!" to the minimum recommended half hour of exercise four to five times each week...

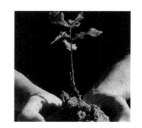

And yet most people would also be surprised by how much exercise they actually do while working in the garden.

So what does gardening have to do with menopause? How can getting mud stuck under your fingernails and fiddling around with tiny seeds enhance your feelings of well-being? Do you mow the lawn? Spend a few hours digging, planting, and/or weeding? Rake the yard? Pick up sticks and loose debris? Well, guess what? That counts as exercise.

What about windy and wet days, when all you want to do is curl up in front of the fire with a romantic novel or a good old black-and-white film and forget what's happening to your body? What if you don't have a garden, or only have a small yard? The answer to all these questions is simple: Go for it and feel better!

Gardening can burn up anywhere between 250 and 400 calories an hour, help keep your bones strong, produce some of your own food, and beat the stress and

Here's an idea for you...

Why not grow nasturtiums in your garden? They look beautiful and you can sprinkle the edible flower petals on your salad.

anxiety you feel when going through menopause. And gardening, especially organic gardening, is not only a way of working up a sweat, but is also a safe and effective way of minimizing many of the changes and symptoms that you will experience during menopause.

These days, women live longer and can look forward to their middle and later years bringing new work, new pastimes and interests, new friendships and relationships. Menopause can be a start to being creatively inspired and productive during this phase. What better way of elevating your moods and relaxing than gardening?

Even if you live in an apartment or have a small patio and don't like the idea of putting yourself on a waiting list to get into a community garden, you can use window boxes or containers that can range from terra-cotta pots to old tires. If you're short of space, you could grow sunflowers and use them as climbing supports for growing snow peas or sunflowers (and you can eat sunflower seeds either raw or after dry roasting them in a hot frying pan). If you like a variety of green leaves in your salad, grow lettuces and spinach. If you want a variety of colors, sprinkle some marigold or wildflower seeds among your vegetables. This will delight your menopausal eye, as it looks pretty and encourages bees to pollinate your plants. Or you could plant chamomile, which not only looks gorgeous but is also long-lasting and even smells beautiful, too.

Create your own space and it will become a place of peace and calm, with wonderful colors and smells. This is the place where you can be alone if you choose, without responsibilities and away from life's daily pressures. Your space will provide you with feelings of refreshment and exhilaration…and this affects your body's levels of serotonin and endorphins, which are the chemicals in the brain that affect your moods. Your own garden can be your tranquil space, used for comfort and revival while you are menopausal, and it's right on your doorstep. And organic gardening increases the chances of small birds, butterflies, and bees visiting your space, bringing you that feeling of fulfillment because you've done it, it's yours.

If you like pleasant smells in your home from your flowers, try the ideas offered in IDEA 27, *It's going on right under your nose.*

Try another idea…

Growing your own organic salad stuff, vegetables, and herbs means that you're eating food that's in as natural a state as possible—and you can season your meals with your homegrown herbs rather than salt. You can save money, pick dinner from your own garden, and get the most delicious fruit and vegetables you've ever tasted—your very own "work of art." The joy of walking out onto your own patch and picking leaves, fruits, and roots to be eaten right away is even greater when you don't have to wash the chemicals off first.

And the science behind it? Lets look at research that's been done already. Dr. Molly Carr, Assistant Professor of Medicine at the University of Washington in Seattle, says, "Women who exercise daily also suffer far fewer severe hot flashes. Menopausal women who are overweight tend to suffer more hot flashes or night sweats than menopausal

"When I go into my garden with a spade, and dig a bed, I feel such an exhilaration and health that I discover that I have been defrauding myself all this time in letting others do for me what I should have done with my own hands."
RALPH WALDO EMERSON

Defining idea…

11

women who aren't." Gardening can produce these improvements. A clinical trial in Germany also confirmed that gardening reduces cholesterol, maintains bone density, and decreases mood swings. So becoming more active results in reducing the need for medication.

Taking up gardening can be a relaxation technique. Being outdoors can be a key aspect of making the transition through menopause simpler and happier. The garden is a place where you can take time for yourself.

How did it go?

Q   I don't have a greenhouse, but I want to grow my own salad stuff. Should I give up?

A   *No, because you really don't need one. There are lots of varieties of tomatoes and cucumbers available that grow outdoors. Visit your local garden center for advice, describing the quality of your soil and the direction your growing plot faces.*

Q   What about slugs and snails? I don't like the idea of killing them with salt and pest controls seem to have chemicals in them.

A   *Sprinkle crushed eggshells around your salad garden...slugs and snails don't like slithering over them!*

4

Picking bones with you

As you reach menopause you can no longer take your bone health for granted.

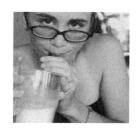

In fact, when you reach your mid-thirties your bones begin to lose density and, unfortunately, start to deteriorate.

Although the basic structure of your bones hasn't changed, they are no longer as strong as they were and are going to need extra support and care to minimize the damage menopause can do to them. What exactly are bones made of, then, and how fast does the deterioration happen?

Well, your bones are composed of the dense outer layer—the cortical bone—which is renewed every twelve years. Then there is the inner trabecular layer, which is renewed every three years; this layer is a softer, spongier bone mass and found in the wrists and hips. (These are the bones most susceptible to breaking, by the way.) Your bones are also made up of collagen and calcium phosphate, and are interspersed with small canals and holes. Bone loss happens when protective levels of estrogen drop and more of these cavities appear, making the bone very fragile.

Here's an idea for you... **Your bones need vitamins B6, C, D, and K, as well as magnesium. Boron, a mineral, is widely believed to be important for menopause and bone loss reduction as well. You might want to consider taking a supplement.**

When bones begin to lose their density they break very easily and as the bone becomes more fragile fractures occur all too easily, as well. Osteoporosis, the name for this loss of bone density, is not painful and can be hard to self-diagnose unless you break a bone, begin to lose height, or have sharp back pain.

You can assess your risk of suffering from osteoporosis by the following:

- Smoking. Smokers are more susceptible to having osteoporosis as smoking can bring about an early menopause, resulting in reduced levels of estrogen production in the body.
- Irregular periods. This can mean you are more at risk because your constant flow of hormones has been interrupted. Women with irregular periods have a lower bone density than those who have regular periods.
- Sedentary lifestyle. Bones need to be worked and need to move. If you spend most of the day sitting down or are bed-ridden, your chances of the disease are higher.

- Lack of sunshine. This means your body is only creating a limited amount of vitamin D, which is vital for bone health.
- Eating disorders. A restricted diet can mean a deficiency in nutrients such as calcium, magnesium, and zinc, which are all vital for bone repair and construction.
- Being underweight. A certain amount of body fat is healthy, especially during menopause when fat cells produce a form of estrogen called estrone.
- Digestive disorders. Celiac disease, Crohn's disease, or some gastric surgery can cause nutrient absorption problems and these can result in osteoporosis.
- A family history of bone degeneration problems. There is a likelihood that osteoporosis is genetic and if you know your mom or dad was a sufferer then you are more at risk.

Although you cannot be sure you will have any problems with your bones it is important that you take the necessary precautions now rather than later. You can make simple but effective changes to your lifestyle and diet to help keep your menopausal bones in tip-top condition.

There are foods you are advised to avoid or limit if you want to reduce the chances of the disease. These are:

For extra useful information about other things to help you with menopause, go to IDEA 31, *Supplements—a waste of money?*

Try another idea…

"I knew a woman, lovely in her bones,
When small birds sighed, she would sigh back at them;
Ah, when she moved, she moved more ways than one;"
THEODORE ROETHKE, poet

Defining idea…

15

- Alcohol
- Animal protein
- Tannins (in tea)
- Salt
- Sodas and sugary drinks

Your daily requirement of calcium will now have increased from 1,000 milligrams to 1,500 milligrams. Dairy foods are not the only source of calcium; some foods such as sesame seeds and herring are also good sources of this vital nutrient. If you eat plenty of fruits and vegetables, you will create good bone mineral density as well as protect against heart disease, and the phytoestrogens in foods such as soy, lentils, and chickpeas all help improve bone density.

Of course, you must make sure your lifestyle includes a regular amount of activity—something that makes your bones work harder than they normally would. Running, skipping, bouncing on a trampoline—or a purpose-made smaller "bouncer"—are all great for preventing osteoporosis.

Q   **I sit at a computer all day, I drive to and from work, and I'm too tired at night to go to an exercise class. How can I minimize my chances of osteoporosis?**

How did it go?

A   *You must do some weight-bearing exercise to put pressure on your bones. Can you make part of your lunch break an active half hour and go for a brisk walk every day? If you do this regularly, it will soon seem very natural— and be so much healthier for you. Go walking whatever the weather so keep galoshes and an umbrella in your car. No excuses.*

Q   **I had a minor fall and was horrified to discover I had actually broken my wrist as a result. I really don't want it to happen again. It was an accident because I tripped over a telephone cord. How can I protect myself against falls?**

A   *Almost all fractures are caused by falls and some of these can definitely be prevented, especially around the home. Everyone needs to be extra careful, not just older people. You must make sure your home is well lit, that all cords are put away, and that you have your eyesight tested regularly. It sounds obvious, but so many homes are rich in opportunities for accidents to happen.*

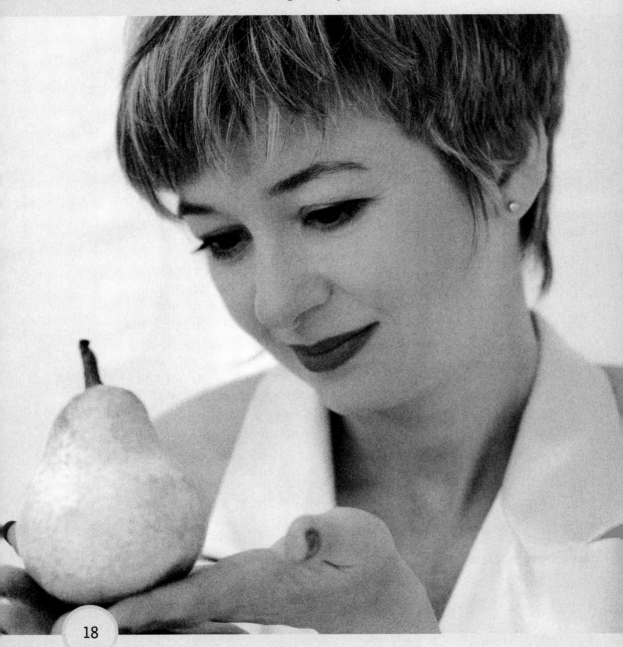

5

Hanging on to your bits and pieces

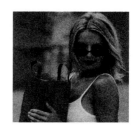

Hair, skin, nails, and teeth...little things like that. Looking good doesn't just happen, and when you're menopausal it can be ten times worse.

Some days you will take one look in the mirror and feel a gloom descend. Right? It takes work—you've got to try your best to keep looking and feeling good.

HAIR

If you are going a menopausal gray in a dull way then don't think twice about getting a color change. Some grays are attractive but others are aging and depressing. Go to a hairdresser and ask for advice. You want a cut you can take care of and a color to mingle with or banish gray hair. Cut out images from magazines, sketch what you have in mind, notice what other women your age are doing with their hair, and go for exactly the cut and style you want.

Try the mini menopausal spa. Facial skin dry? Mix four tablespoons of olive oil with some Dead Sea salts and gently scrub any patchy, rough areas of flaky skin. Rinse off using a clean washcloth soaked in warm water to open your pores, and then open a vitamin E capsule and gently massage the oil onto your face.

Menopause might have left you with thinning hair, so if you notice a few extra hairs on the pillow in the morning then make sure you are downing the right amounts of essential fatty acids (omega-3 and omega-6), such as those found in fish and olive oil. Spinach, high in the super B vitamins, beats hair loss and the B group might also slow down or prevent your hair from graying. Follow a diet enriched with fresh foods—live yogurts, organic vegetables and fruits, figs, dates, legumes—to give your hair the very best chance in life.

SKIN

Most women suffer from dry skin during menopause and a good moisturizer is worth its weight in gold. You'll need different skin care products now, so always ask for samples and freebies until you discover the best ones for you. Practice a regular skin care routine each evening and every morning:

- Cleanse thoroughly
- Exfoliate regularly to slough off dead cells
- Tone to calm the skin
- Apply moisturizer

Your skin will respond to being fed and watered on the inside, too. Drinking regular glasses of water throughout the day will help to keep your skin plumped up and smooth. Vitamin B$_2$ and riboflavin, which is found in avocados, will help repair cracked and very dry skin. Avocados also contain vitamin E and will protect your skin against menopausal aging. Watercress, a good source of antioxidants, will help clean up those free radicals your skin might have been exposed to in the sun.

Check out IDEA 32, *It's her hormones...*, for information about hormones and how they affect your body.

Try another idea…

NAILS

You've probably never worn rubber gloves when doing housework but they are a must if you want to protect your nails from the harsh chemicals found in most domestic cleansers. Hot, soapy water isn't good for your nails as it makes them weak and soft, so wear those rubber gloves. Use a barrier cream every time your hands have been in water and apply nail oil and cuticle treatment oil a couple of times a week to let your nails have the best chance of firming up, and to prevent splitting. A regular manicure is both a good tonic and relaxing, which is great for everything.

Weak nails often indicate a calcium deficiency—common during menopause—so increase your calcium intake by eating more cheese, spinach, parsley, watercress, nuts, and dried figs. Little white spots are a sign of zinc deficiency. Zinc is found in oysters, red meat, beans, grains, and tofu, and you may

"The body is a sacred garment. It's your first and last garment: it is what you enter life in and what you depart life with, and it should be treated with honor."
MARTHA GRAHAM

Defining idea…

21

need to supplement your diet, especially if you are vegetarian. White-lined bands can signal protein deficiency. You can remedy this by eating protein-rich nuts, eggs, dairy products, lean meat—and vitamin B_{12} strengthens and protects nail growth.

TEETH

If you have any issues with your teeth—gaps or fillings that need replacing—then now is a good time to get them fixed. A healthy mouth and a set of teeth you are proud of will both help boost your morale. You could also try out those tongue scrapers and use one to help eliminate any bacteria gathered in your mouth before you start brushing your teeth with a scrupulously clean toothbrush.

Make sure you eat plenty of calcium-rich foods such as green leafy vegetables and salmon, and drinking a tablespoon of cider vinegar each day in a cup of warm water with honey will help your body absorb calcium more easily. Vitamin C is important for gums and teeth but beware of taking too much; it's very acid-forming and this in turn will cause damage to your teeth and encourage calcium loss.

Finally, though prevention is always better than cure, it isn't the end of the world if you do need any teeth removed. Modern dentistry offers fabulous alternatives to those dentures your grandma had.

Q **I seem to have aged since menopause began. My facial bone structure isn't particularly strong. Is there anything I can do?**

How did it go?

A *Collagen is a natural protein that gives the body shape and texture. As we age the collagen breaks down and is not replaced, so a collagen deficiency will show up as wrinkles and saggy skin. A good collagen cream or serum will help firm and plump facial tissue and help smooth away wrinkles.*

Q **When I started menopause the skin on my feet seemed to become very tough and dry. What's the best thing to do?**

A *Use a foot file to remove all dead and hard skin every day, before you take a bath or shower. Then apply a foot cream—this will keep your feet soft and smooth and prevent a buildup of further hard skin.*

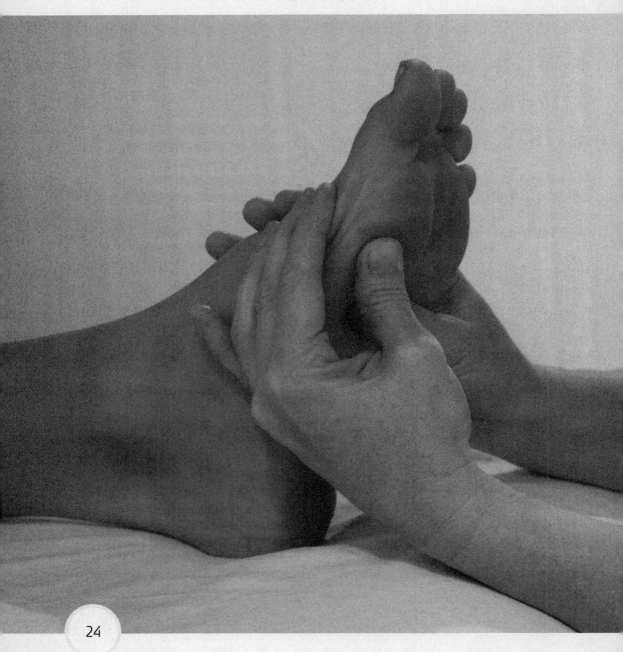

6

Give yourself a good going-over

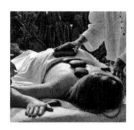

Massage is nothing new. Touch is one of the earliest forms of healing, and sometimes just the lightest touch can say more than a thousand words.

It can be a wonderful antidote to the pressures in your hectic life.

You know what it's like when you are feeling tired and someone just rubs your shoulder or pats you on the back. It can make all the difference to your sense of well-being. It's not always possible to get to a salon and the chances of being able to get a masseur to your home are probably as impossible as they are impractical. Well, you know what they say: If you want a job done right, do it yourself.

When you are menopausal, massage is a lifesaver and can make you feel relaxed, back in control, and able to face the day again. When you are stressed and weary with menopausal symptoms you can become tense, and these feelings of tension can impair the proper circulation of blood and oxygen to the muscles and organs. This can cause feelings of tiredness, fatigue, and lethargy. When you are active and on top of things, your lymphatic system is working wonders maintaining and regulating your body's fluid balance. As soon as you feel stressed and your muscles

Here's an idea for you... **Use a tennis ball to help you unwind and make it your menopausal ally. How? By lying on the floor with the tennis ball tucked under your back. Relax as you roll around on it and you'll feel it work wonders in relieving tension.**

tighten, this ceases and the lymphatic system isn't as effective, so waste and toxins begin to store up and make you feel worse.

This is never more apparent than when you are menopausal. I regularly visit a friend who is also menopausal and she has a hugely hectic lifestyle—teenage children at home, a successful shop to run—and she loves nothing more than a massage. But she dislikes going to a salon because she has all the trouble of undressing, then dressing again, then going home to cooking, kids, and the phone ringing every two minutes. We devised a plan whereby she would let me have a lovely item from her store in exchange for a massage. It worked wonders, but for the days we can't see each other we both use the self-massage technique. Through regular self-massage you will be in charge of your own well-being, as well as develop a systematic approach to self-healing. So on those days that menopause is driving you up the wall, or you are in need of some TLC, or you need to access some hidden energy, you can get right to it. Here's how.

After a stressful day, chances are you are all wrinkled and furrowed. Here is a way to rid yourself of the worst of these lines:

- Using your fingertips, apply firm pressure, taking care not to drag the skin but to manipulate the tissue beneath the skin's surface, and begin with the forehead.
- Apply pressure to the center of the forehead and now work your hands to the sides of your face. Repeat this a few times before moving your fingertips across your cheekbones and finally over your whole face.

- Repeat this until you feel a glow of warmth spread across your face and your shoulders begin to drop as well.

Try IDEA 9, *All that posturing*, for more self-help healing habits.

Try another idea...

Next, use a slapping technique. This is one we used as a warm-up when I worked in theater and it really did stimulate a marvelous tingling sensation and sense of a waking up and alertness:

- Using your fingers, loosely tap your all over head.
- Move down to your neck, chest, and shoulders and feel the slaps become tighter as you close your fingers and looser as you open them more.
- Continue down your legs, really slapping those thighs. Go right down your legs to your feet.

If you have one of those menopausal headaches coming on, then this technique should relieve the pressure:

- Put your fingertips against the scalp along your hairline.
- Apply pressure to the scalp and release. Apply and release.
- Once you have done this a few times gently pull at clumps of hair—just enough to feel it and let go. Breathe in as you pull and out as you release.

"Have a heart that never hardens, and a temper that never tires, and a touch that never hurts."

CHARLES DICKENS

Defining idea...

Finally, to relieve a tense neck, try this:

- Put both hands on your shoulders and pull your hands down, allowing your head to fall backward slowly and carefully.
- Feel each muscle in your shoulder as you do it.

27

Do these five or six times. Don't they allow you to feel where the knots are? So if you can't get to a masseur there's no need to fret: You have the world at your fingertips.

How did
it go?

Q   I can't go for a daily massage but feel I need something to help my aching joints. The mornings are worst. Can you suggest anything?

A   *An acupressure expert I contacted suggested you try massaging your toes like this: Take one toe at a time and gently twist the joints in each toe. Massage and twist the entire foot area. This action helps with joint mobility and should ease discomfort if done every day.*

Q   I feel such tightness during the night when I wake up in a sweat, thanks to menopause. What relief is there for me?

A   *For tightness and a need to cool off a bit, you could put a wet towel in the freezer. When you wake up, take it out and apply it to your neck. It will alleviate the heat as well as remove stiffness from your neck. Moreover, it is surprising how quickly the towel warms up with your own body heat. This sounds worse than it actually is!*

7

It's not all black and white

Can color make a difference during menopause?

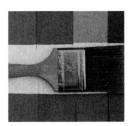

The answer is simply YES! Color is everywhere, in everything you do, see, touch, or eat. You cannot escape your involvement with color...even when you sleep.

When you are balanced, you can more effectively fight illnesses and rid your system of toxins, as well as negative energy. This balance, so important for your menopausal years, can be achieved through color.

How? Well, color can affect your energy in a way that stabilizes your physical, emotional, mental, and spiritual conditions. You've seen the ads on TV by paint companies; you're told colors relate to your moods. Yet, quite apart from the beauty of those colors you like, using colors can relieve the stresses and anxieties caused by menopause. Colors let you express yourself, can reveal how you feel about yourself and how others see you. You are affected by different colored light and even by the colors you wear. Color is used to calm and to balance...it is even used in therapies. Here is a simple guide to some colors and their meanings:

Here's an idea for you...

Try visualizing color when you are having an "off" menopausal moment and everything is getting you down. Take a few deep breaths, close your eyes, and flood your mind with a color you know makes you feel restored and peaceful again. It's a lovely pick-me-up.

Red gives us courage, strength, and relates to stability and security. Red is the symbol of love and anger and life itself, and it generates enthusiasm, arouses passion, and has a cheering effect.

Blue is a cooling, soothing color used to increase vitality and energy, so it can help relieve menopausal difficulties and nervous irritability. Blue has a calming effect, so it is very helpful with sleep disorders and headaches. Blue represents the spirit of purpose and truth.

Yellow is a clear purifying color, which stimulates our clarity of meaning. Yellow is the color of joy, it helps to soothe the emotions and relieve depression. Use yellow for mental fatigue and for stimulating activity, so poor concentration may be improved by yellows. Yellow can act as a stimulator and balancer of the nervous system.

Violet is one of the "cool" colors. It has a very calming effect on us and is helpful when experiencing stress or sleep difficulties. Violet relates to self-knowledge and spiritual awareness. It increases the benefits of meditation, and is very helpful during menopause. It is the color for neutralizing emotional wounds and for spiritual growth.

Green is the color of energy and youth. Green can stimulate the nervous system and soothe the emotions. It is used to treat irritability, menopausal sleeplessness, and nervous disorders. Green is a cooling color, which helps calm the body. It's the color of the relaxed heart.

Orange is the color of creativity. Your creativity is enhanced during menopause, so give yourself the space to have creative time just for you. Orange symbolizes joy and happiness and helps raise the spirit. It promotes a healthy appetite and increases the sex drive. It's a bright and warm source of encouragement for all aspects of life.

Go to IDEA 38, *Looking back to the future*, for ways to remember a colorful past.

Try another idea…

Turquoise is the color for mental relaxation and tackling embedded psychological barriers. It tones and can help regulate imbalances. It is a color that facilitates spiritual growth.

You can decorate your home to take advantage of the properties of color. For example, a plain white quilt cover, a glittering crystal light fitting, or a new set of crushed silk rose-pink curtains can have a very positive and powerful impact and make a great deal of difference to your mood. Choose colors after a few trials, and don't rush into using any color until you have tested it and seen how it makes you feel. Some can seem like a great idea until you've got a headache and realize too late that the color you used in your bedroom isn't helping you feel better, and could even be making you feel worse.

Defining idea…

"We are energy, we are color. When we are out of balance, there can be too much or too little of a color in us, and this in time will manifest itself as a disease. By introducing a specific color as vibrational energy, we can harmonize disorders within the body and improve physical, mental, emotional, and spiritual health."
RENEE GANGER, color therapist

Here are a few other simple suggestions of how you can use color in your home:

- Use colored lamps or buy colored bulbs.
- Use soft lights instead of fluorescent or neon.
- Use gentle and harmonious shades.

31

- Carefully choose the colors you use—whether this is for your clothes, home furnishings, or bedroom.
- Use natural colors. These are the most beneficial, nourishing, and strengthening. Think about those colors that appear naturally: in the sky, the sea, in the natural landscape including trees, flowers, or fields.

How did it go?

Q   What about clothes? My taste seems to be changing... Can I still wear the colors I want?

A   *Yes! Just remember you will find yourself wearing clothes that reflect your moods and the color of the clothes you wear can alter the way you feel. The colors you wear can directly relate to the way you feel in your menopausal cycle. For example, wear bright clothes to counter depression or a lack of self-confidence, or wear calming colors to suppress irritability or stress, often symptoms of menopause.*

Q   I don't want to sound silly, but what about the color of food? Does it matter what color food is while I'm menopausal?

A   *Yes, it does. Food affects your moods and the color of food is very important. You can even eat appropriately colored food to match your mood. Vary your diet according to how you feel or how you want to feel. For example, think about yellow foods such as bananas or sweet corn, green salad leaves, red tomatoes, strawberries... There's lots of potential.*

8

Moving mountains

Who wants to exercise when it's cold, rainy, and there's a good film on TV? But exercise is extremely important now that you are in menopause.

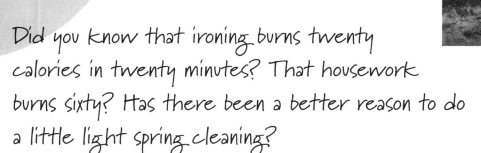

Did you know that ironing burns twenty calories in twenty minutes? That housework burns sixty? Has there been a better reason to do a little light spring cleaning?

Regular exercise not only benefits your heart and bones and helps regulate your weight, but it also contributes to your sense of overall well-being and improvement in mood. The good news is that a regular program of physical activity can help manage many of the uncomfortable symptoms of menopause as well as the related health concerns, such as heart disease and osteoporosis. During exercise, hormones called endorphins are released into your brain. These make doing that little bit of exercise all the more worthwhile. You get a real high and the "feel-good" factor is your body's positive response to stress.

In other words, a good bout of moving at a good pace somehow can work wonders for the way we menopausal women feel. Right? I hate to admit it, but it's true. I'm always happy I've done it—after the event. But I still always dread it just before, and still look for excuses not to walk but to take the car.

Here's an idea for you… **Instead of parking your car in your work garage, try parking it twenty minutes or so away from your workplace so you have to walk the rest of the way. You will soon get used to it and it means you are exercising every day for at least forty minutes.**

Aerobic exercise also helps you shift that roll of tummy fat—the place you have probably noticed you've been piling it on since menopause started. That news can only make you feel better as well, can't it? In addition, some research studies have shown that the increased estrogen levels that follow a woman's exercise session coincide with an overall decrease in the severity of hot flashes…and that has to be a good thing, too.

WAYS YOU CAN EXERCISE

Walking is a great way, is cheap, and can be done without any serious preparation and in all weather. Try walking for at least an hour, four or five times every week. Weight-bearing exercise using weights, or resistance bands and flexibility, is essential. You can also run, skip, or play tennis to get the same effect. Yoga will keep you flexible and supple in both mind and body. Swimming is good for stamina, an overall sense of well-being, and mobility.

Although gym membership can be prohibitively expensive, many gyms offer the opportunity to attend classes without joining on an annual basis. These classes can be taken whenever you have the time and may include salsa dancing, fat burning, kickboxing, and circuit training among many others. They are great fun and you won't feel intimidated or embarrassed to go to these as the "body beautifuls" tend to be in the gym itself wearing headphones and watching weird TV channels as they cycle their way to thinness.

MORE WAYS IT HELPS

Now this part is impressive. Exercise helps with menopause in so many ways it's crazy not to try it. Exercise will:

See IDEA 4, *Picking bones with you*, for ways of keeping your bones in the best of health.

Try another idea…

- Improve function of the immune and lymphatic systems as well as keep your blood sugar levels in balance
- Provide strength, stamina, flexibility, energy
- Maintain the function of vital organs
- Maintain bone and muscle density
- Maintain and improve the condition of your heart, lungs, and muscles
- Prevent hot flashes
- Prevent vaginal and bladder atrophy
- Ease joint pain
- Prevent heart disease
- Prevent osteoporosis
- Prevent weight gain
- Relieve anxiety, irritability, and depression
- Relieve sleep disturbances and insomnia

Finally, there are the energy boosts you get from making love, laughing, decorating the house, and gardening. Take the stairs wherever possible and make that heart pump for you; you'll soon get the hang of it and the elevator will become a dirty word. There are so many ways to get your body moving again. Plus, each time you get some exercise you know you are doing something positive toward menopause. Trust me—I'm out there with you.

"I don't exercise. If God had wanted me to bend over, he would have put diamonds on the floor."

JOAN RIVERS

Defining idea…

35

How did
it go?

Q **I hate exercising and, although I am menopausal, I am not over-weight so I don't really see the need to go to a gym. But I would like to do something active for my well-being. Any suggestions?**

A *Take something new, a class you have never tried before, and that way you won't get bored—try a rock and roll dance class or even tap dancing. You will be strengthening all your muscles as well as increasing vitality levels and coordination.*

Q **I have a bike and would love to get it out again but feel like such a fool cycling with one of those helmets on, and wouldn't be seen dead with my menopausal rear in those Lycra shorts. How can I get the best from my bike if it just sits in the garage rusting away?**

A *Cycling is such a good exercise but I know what you mean about feeling self-conscious. Also I am not convinced the roads in cities and towns are safe for cyclists. But if you really want to get out and about on your bike I suggest you ask a friend or member of your family to get a bike as well and go off for a day somewhere. You could get off the beaten track, stop for lunch—a salad, of course—and then cycle home. It's a great way to see the countryside and you won't be driven half mad by stressed-out motorists. Make a day of it and you will feel reenergized, exercised, relaxed, and you won't have given a second thought to your menopause.*

9

All that posturing

Pilates is big business...

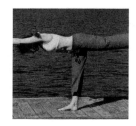

...and it's little wonder that Elizabeth Hurley and Sarah Jessica Parker are huge advocates of the exercise system designed to correct body alignment.

Joseph Pilates, a German physical-fitness trainer, skier, gymnast, and wrestler, designed this program of movements with menopause in mind. Well, so it seems. Born in 1880, Pilates wanted to sculpt his naturally wispy body so he studied everything from boxing, skiing, and fencing to swimming, until at the age of about fourteen he was working as a male model for anatomical drawings.

What does that have to do with menopause?

Well, Pilates believed that instead of doing a series of repetitive movements to build up muscle mass, a more focused, concentrated, conscious flow of actions would be advantageous. The method he designed is the concentrated use of your mind and body to get the body you want. That's what makes it special. It uses a holistic approach and you work with your body, not against it. When you are menopausal you have enough battles, and psychologically it is beneficial to approach your body

Here's an idea for you…

Make sure you have a solid mattress because how you sleep on it will give you a good spinal alignment and straighten your spine while you sleep. A decent mattress is a sound investment, especially through menopause when sleeping might be a challenge for you anyway. Try the mattresses out in the store and go for the best you can afford.

as an ally and not an enemy. Also, when menopause strikes and estrogen levels drop, you can be susceptible to bone loss. This is apparent at the top of the spine—you might have seen women with a curvature sometimes associated with menopause, a condition called kyphosis. It can be helped with Pilates.

Pilates believed you should always be clear about how and why you are moving your body. The system is based on six main principles:

1. Concentration
2. Control
3. Centering
4. Flow
5. Precision
6. Breath

You do Pilates by:

- Lengthening short muscles and strengthening weak ones
- Controlling your smallest movements
- Improving the way you move
- Breathing correctly

- Mentally relaxing as you move
- Focusing on core muscles to stabilize your body

During menopause Pilates can help you with:

- Increasing your flexibility
- Improving your posture
- Improving your muscle tone
- Increasing your stamina
- Improving your circulation and respiration
- Increasing your bone density
- Increasing your energy levels
- Boosting your immune system
- Increasing your sense of well-being
- Reducing stress levels
- Strengthening pelvic floor muscles

Good posture makes you feel taller and slimmer; it helps you create an air of confidence about yourself, something you might need through menopause. And better posture helps you to be noticed: One thing some people worry about is that they seem to have become invisible. Good posture can also help you sleep better; it decreases the wear and tear on your ligaments and so prevents arthritis.

Try IDEA I, _Bent double_, to help you discover ways to let added suppleness help your posture and movement.

Try another idea...

"There are thoughts which are prayers. There are moments when, whatever the posture of your body, the soul is on its knees."

VICTOR HUGO

Defining idea...

Pilates can help you find a good sitting position. Sit at the end of your chair and slouch completely, then draw yourself up and accentuate the curve of your back as far as possible. Hold for a few seconds. Now release the position slightly (about ten degrees). This is a good sitting posture. Distribute your body weight evenly on both hips. Bend your knees at a right angle. Keep your knees even with, or slightly higher than, your hips (use a footrest or stool if necessary). Your legs should not be crossed. Keep your feet flat on the floor. Try to avoid sitting in the same position for more than thirty minutes.

At work, adjust your chair height and workstation so you can sit close to your work and tilt it up at you. Rest your elbows and arms on your chair or desk, keeping your shoulders relaxed. When sitting in a chair that rolls and pivots, do not twist at the waist while sitting; instead, turn your whole body. When standing up from the sitting position, move to the front of the seat of your chair and stand up by straightening your legs. Avoid bending forward at the waist.

Q Since menopause, I have become somewhat overweight and I
have noticed a roll of fat around my middle and cannot shift this.
I spend most of my day standing and think this might be making
my condition worse. What do you think?

*How did
it go?*

A *You definitely need some posture programming, as this will only become
more severe with age. Your weight means you have been counterbalanc-
ing yourself and have produced very rigid spinal "erectors." This means
your front side is weaker now. To remedy this, you must stand correctly.
You need to stand with your feet hip-width apart, with both feet facing
forward. Don't lock your knees but let them relax and soften a little. Allow
your arms to rest by your side and feel your weight being supported by the
middle of each foot. Do not rock back but allow the balls of your feet to
carry your weight.*

Q I seem to be hunched up all day, especially after a bad night's
sleep. Menopause can keep me awake for hours and then I think
I sleep in a bad position so my body feels very uncomfortable
when I wake up. How can I make a better routine a habit so that I
allow my body to unfold a little?

A *The moment you wake up have a great big yawn. Then stretch your arms
and legs as you lie in bed. Stretching will help you lengthen your muscles
and relieve any muscle tension you have accumulated through the night.
Before you get out of bed, curl up like a cat and slowly uncurl. You will
probably feel your spine coming to life again. Do this four or five times.*

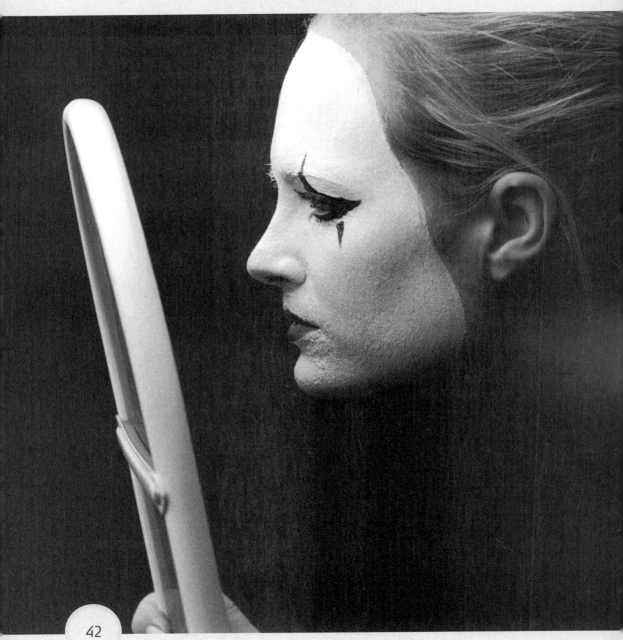

10

Am I still attractive?

Menopause can make you doubt that you are still a desirable woman. The fact is that the opposite is true. You are highly desirable and remarkably attractive.

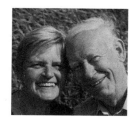

It's more than understandable to doubt your own beauty as a woman when you are menopausal...

The media is full of images of half-naked, young, skinny women and, if that's not bad enough, the other images are of celebrities up to their eyeballs in cosmetic surgery. For the likes of you and me getting by on a few creams, lotions, and a lot of prayer, it does seem a bit unfair.

On top of that, you might find that you are losing interest in sex and suddenly a week, a month, and then a year can pass and you haven't been making love. As soon as you get out of practice of making love for a while, self-doubt sets in and you begin to wonder whether you're desirable. You might not want to talk about it at all but, on the other hand, you might find yourself yelling at your lover about the lack of action in the bedroom department...then your partner retaliates by blaming you, and it all becomes a mess. By the time you hit the sack neither of you are talking. How does it get to that point?

Here's an idea for you...

If you've recently relied on pornography to help you along then this might be the time to get back to basics and ditch it. Tempt each other with nothing more than your own bodies. It might be a bit of a problem to begin with, but by letting go of the porn you will soon enough reaffirm your lust and desire for each other. Create a storm in your bedroom "as nature intended" and you'll reap the rewards when the passion and love for each other floods back again.

I know that you might be tired, fed up, and feeling quite unsexy—and that little list is more than enough of a reason not to make love. But most women, menopausal or not, enjoy making love. It is a way of expressing not only feelings of love for another human being, but of giving yourselves time to enjoy each other.

It's too easy for lovers to drift into becoming a couple who, at every bedtime, give a little peck on the cheek and read a good book before turning over and falling asleep. It does seem like a waste when you could be having a really good time together—not every night, perhaps, but a couple of times a month can't be out of the question, can it? I hear so many women "joke" that their guys are no longer interested in them and don't do anything with them anymore. Fix it! There is only one way to find out what the problem is and that is to ask. It could be a health issue, a fear of impotence, or any number of things. But as soon as you know you can talk about it, then you can do something about it.

WHAT YOU CAN DO

A massage might get you interested in making physical contact with your partner again, as might lying in front of the fire naked together. If you miss the little sex rituals you had, then reintroduce them into your life. Have sex on the sofa while the television is on. Maybe during the big game is pushing things a bit far, but if you're feeling particularly brave you could give it a try.

Take your time and feel confident in your ability to take some responsibility for the way you feel—and look. Become interested in yourself and your appearance again. When you "feel" your beauty yourself, then your partner certainly will.

To understand what might be going on with your sexual anatomy, see IDEA 28, *OH OH OH OH...oh?*, to keep you informed.

Try another idea...

ANYTHING ELSE?

Get to know each other again. Book a hotel room for the two of you and ask to have breakfast in bed. If you want to, hang a "Do Not Disturb" sign on the door and stay in bed the whole weekend. Go sightseeing and relax together. Just having time and no agenda, other than to have no agenda, is wonderful. So many couples I know don't take any time out together and then complain that they are frazzled, constantly arguing, and feel life is passing them by. There is nothing nicer than rediscovering your lover and becoming interested in each other all over again.

"The real voyage of discovery consists not in seeking new landscapes but in having new eyes."

MARCEL PROUST

Defining idea...

Q   I admit I have let myself go a little but to be honest I don't care. I don't want sex again and I don't miss it. Is there something wrong with me?

A   *There is a relationship between how you feel about yourself and your sex drive. The better you feel about how you look and how healthy you are the more it seems to trigger a sexual appetite again. Once you have got yourself feeling and looking tip-top again you'll be surprised at how quickly your sex life will be restored.*

Q   I am very tempted to have an affair. My husband and I used to have a great sex life but haven't been near each other for ages. A man at work has shown great interest in me and I like the attention. Should I go for it?

A   *Obviously you don't need permission from anyone to start an affair but it is wise to consider what you might be throwing away if you do embark on one. If you don't know why you and your husband have stopped making love then it might be a better idea to focus on the relationship you have instead of starting a new one. If you cannot fix things with your partner and if it seems as though there is no love between you then obviously you will have to consider splitting up with him and find a new soul mate. But affairs while married rarely work out in a satisfactory way for anyone.*

11

Picture this...

"Where attention goes, energy flows." I know you've been there, done that, and got a few T-shirts. This time make a decision to believe in what you are doing.

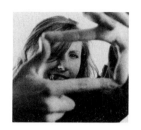

Creative visualization works for plenty of people; it could work for you as well.

Your imagination is incredibly powerful and, when used correctly, can enhance your life by helping you create a better relationship with your body now that you are in menopause. Learning to use your imagination in a conscious way is a creative tool you can use every single day and it will:

- Reduce your menopausal anxiety, depression, stress, and mood swings.
- Increase mental stamina, improving your memory, focus, and multitasking abilities.
- Break through long-standing blocks to your well-being, spiritual growth, and communication as well as your overall relationship health.
- Give a feeling of deep calm.

During menopause things will happen all the time that are beyond your control, but it is how you respond to the situation that counts. These so-called negative experiences or problems are excellent opportunities to change the way you think and behave. When you begin to have control over the way you can direct your

Here's an idea for you...

When you are struggling with disappointment and can't quite find the energy to get over it, take a few minutes to think back to a time you fought for something and won. This can be called your "warrior" energy and will help you through menopause. Make a little symbol of your warrior and keep it somewhere you can refer to when you feel you might be particularly vulnerable.

imagination to create positive change, then your nervous system begins to reap the rewards. Your brain chemistry becomes balanced, creating a sense of well-being and happiness, something you definitely need during menopause. So let's get going.

Ensure you are seated comfortably, with no possible interruptions, and clear your mind of any thoughts. As your mind becomes clear, begin to imagine that all the physical menopausal stresses have been removed from your body. During your deep exhales of breath imagine the stress and tension has been expelled from your body and has disintegrated in the air. As you are visualizing this stress leaving you, begin to feel your body becoming more relaxed.

Next, relax each part of your body in turn, beginning with your toes and moving upward or starting with your head and moving down. Now center your awareness by breathing slowly and then, as you exhale, imagine you are breathing out through a spot just below your navel. Place your hand on your tummy to keep your awareness there.

Focus on the relaxed state of your body and say an affirmation that will enhance this process, such as something like:

- I am now in a totally relaxed state.
- My mind is now clear and my body has released all the stresses and tension.

Go to IDEA 18, *Ever been needled?*, for added awareness about how to stimulate energies in your body and mind.

Try another idea...

See yourself as you would like to be in a few months time—very much enjoying menopause and creating feelings of warmth and happiness around you. See yourself as the powerful woman who has begun to meet her needs and is having all of them met. See yourself as being wise, creative, in touch with what is going on in the world and see yourself helping effect change somewhere in the world, no matter how small.

How do you want to look in menopause? How do you want to sound, feel, and smell? See a total picture of the woman you are and see menopause as being instrumental in helping rather than hindering you in getting what you want. Have total faith that what you see is as real as the room you are in.

Now decide quite clearly what else you need to bring about your ideal life. This could include:

- A closer relationship
- A more vibrant life
- A more fulfilling career

You decide and don't worry if you want lots of changes; you can ask for as many as you want.

"An affirmation is a strong, positive statement that something is already so."
SHAKTI GAWAIN, author

Defining idea...

49

Once you have seen yourself in this new role really breathe in the woman you want to be as though she is already with you. Then make it "real": Put pen to paper and write out your ideal scenario in the present tense as though you have already achieved what you want. Use your imagination to the fullest to completely describe how you saw yourself, your surroundings, clothes, lifestyle, and career. Most important of all, write down how you felt about menopause in this ideal state.

How did it go?

Q **As soon as menopause started I began making creative visualization a weekly activity. But should I be doing it every day?**

A *Yes, it would help you immerse yourself in the positive landscape you want to create for yourself if you make it a daily practice. You can do it anywhere—but once a week make a special time to review your visualizations and anything you might want to change, as well as make a note of developments in your life (they will happen).*

Q **My husband thinks I am involved with witchcraft because I spend time each night visualizing by candlelight. I think it's really helped me with menopause but he thinks it's all garbage. How can I get him to join in?**

A *Could you point out to him where the best changes in your life are happening and how they were all visualized by you before they happened? Get him to join in, but in a lighthearted way, and see if he finds it relaxing—then he might enjoy it and make it permanent.*

12

What do you mean you "feel like a woman"?

Some men find it hard to cope with their partner's menopause and this can mean that we turn to other women who are more understanding.

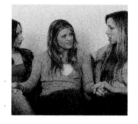

And it is true that some women do become interested in other women once menopause starts. No need to panic, fret, or consider a sex change.

If you start to become uninterested in sex or withdraw more and find it hard to respond if your partner reaches out to touch you, it can mean the relationship is in trouble. If your partner has spent years using you for sex—for his own pleasure, without considering whether you were ready for sex or even wanted sex or not—then now that you are in menopause it is highly likely you will react differently and mean it when you say "no more." But it can be a sad and lonely time if you feel you can't or don't want to express your feelings about the relationship.

Here's an idea for you… **Forget "girlie" nights—go for the real thing and have "women" nights where you can meet up regularly and talk about your relationships, men, films, books, politics—anything you want. Make the evening really enjoyable: Eat, drink, and track each other's progress. Then if something goes wrong, you have a network of people ready to offer you their advice, love, and encouragement.**

If you have stopped having fun, or you no longer laugh or share intimate moments together, you might feel desperate to talk to someone about what you are going through. It might not be your partner's fault, of course; it could be that you have raised the bar and that your expectations of what makes a relationship nurturing and satisfying have changed.

Talk to your female friends about their relationships—where they work, what they still want from these relationships, and why they might not be as rewarding as they had hoped. What did they do when their relationships went through rocky patches? Have your women friends ever stopped having sex with men and, if so, what did they do about it? What they say could have some bearing on your own life.

If your partner won't or can't talk about deeply personal things to you then it could be that you turn to a woman for a relationship. It can happen around menopause. In addition, your sexual orientation may have shifted with menopause, and what used to satisfy you sexually no longer does. If you have had a sexual liaison with a woman in the past, you could find yourself fantasizing about her at this time. Maybe even more than fantasizing, perhaps actually seeking her out or looking for another woman to love in a passionate relationship. A woman might be exactly what you need at this time to take you to a place of tenderness, warmth, and sexual expression.

It doesn't have to be physical; it could be that a very close and loving but non-sexual relationship with a woman is just what you need. Make your friendships with women close and tight. Listen to them and talk to your friends "soul to soul." Menopause offers you the chance to view women in a very different light. Until now you might never have noticed how wonderfully sexy and funny older women are. You know now what other women have gone through and are going through. You know them to be caring, spiritual, wise, and earthy, intuitive, intelligent, and attractive.

All relationships, whatever the sex of the other person involved, suffer the same emotional roller coaster of jealousies, anger, and fear. All relationships need an airing out, especially when menopause comes along to rock the boat and possibly steer you off in different directions.

It's a good idea to become more involved with women of every age. Read up on IDEA 50, *Gorgeous, sexy, and I hate you!*, to find out why.

Try another idea…

"I have lived and slept in the same bed as English countesses and Prussian farm women…no woman has excited passions more than I have."

FLORENCE NIGHTINGALE

Defining idea…

53

How did it go?

Q **My husband works late, the children have left home, and I am feeling desperately lonely. I have lost touch with my old friends and would really like to see some women for nights out and fun again. What should I do?**

A *Tell your husband how you are feeling. Ask him what he thinks of your relationship and whether there is any point in continuing a relationship with so little interaction. If he wants it to work then he is going to have to make sure he contributes more fully—in every way—than he is now. Meanwhile, why not log on to a social networking site, find your old friends again, and enjoy being with people who knew you from the past? When you make a first move to become proactive, friends will come swarming into your life.*

Q **I am about to leave my husband for a woman I knew when I was in my twenties. My partner knows about it but I am terrified of telling my children, even though they are adults. Should I tell them before I leave?**

A *You must let them know as soon as possible so they have a chance to let you know how they feel. If you leave it until you have moved in with your new partner it will be too late for them to feel they have had your trust. You should wait until you have told them before introducing your new partner to them. Try to minimize any pain. Tell them your feelings have changed, but stress that it's not because of them.*

13

"Er, what was I saying?"

You've done it again: walked into the boss's office and, midsentence, had no idea what you were going to say.

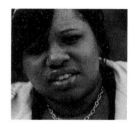

You make a fumbling excuse and head for the door when you suddenly remember why you went in there in the first place and have to go back.

Memory loss is one of the effects of a drop in estrogen levels at menopause and it can be infuriating to feel efficient and composed one minute and like a gibbering idiot the next. It might be amusing once or twice, but after that it can be a totally humiliating experience.

Before you do anything else you need to make sure you are aware, totally aware, every minute of the day, that you have the potential to forget anything and everything.

You might already be writing things down on pieces of paper by the phone but then you lose that paper and spend half an hour trying to find it. So, one good thing

Here's an idea for you... **Although you can multitask till the cows come home and might seem to spend your days making all those mental notes of what needs to be done at home, at work, at play, you still need time to stop and unwind. Instead of watching television, take fifteen minutes out to relax and listen to beautiful music, a relaxation tape, or simply wallow in silence. It really will be worth those fifteen minutes for the peace of mind this brings.**

to do is to carry around a very firm notepad or small book, and make this notebook your real friend. It will definitely help you out to no end. Write things down. Within a short period, the act of doing this will become second nature to you, so make a note of everything that you need to do. This will free you up to do the more important things in your life.

To help you feel in control it might help if you empty out your handbag at the end of each day. Make sure it holds only what you need for the following day. It's awful to spend time rummaging through a bag crammed with old receipts, train tickets, makeup, a letter you forgot to mail, and all the other stuff we carry around every day. Pull out the junk and trash it. If you carry "light," and only take what you know you'll need, you will feel so much more organized. If you can leave the house and go to work after a calm start—instead of all frazzled having spent an hour hunting for the car keys—you'll arrive much more capable of coping with the demands of the day.

It can be useful to try something I was told recently and that is to give yourself an aural message about where you have put something. For instance, if you leave your car at the end of Level 4 in the parking garage, next to the blue exit door, then actually say it out loud. Say "I'm leaving my car at the far end of the parking garage on Level 4 by the blue exit door." It's another way to reinforce the memory; by saying it you will recall what you told yourself and no longer have to hunt around for things.

If you want some extra help with sorting out and clearing up go to IDEA 21, *Space Clearing.*

Try another idea…

CAN I TAKE ANYTHING TO HELP?

Make sure you take a good multivitamin and mineral supplement during this time as well as boosting your intake of the phytoestrogen found in soy, which should help you with your memory. Ginkgo biloba is also beneficial for the brain, nerves, and blood vessels. Its reputation as an "anti-aging" herb seems to be appropriate. Its effects on memory, brain function, and circulation have made this venerable tree one of the most extensively studied and widely used botanicals in the world. Strong clinical evidence shows that it can help improve declining brain function in elderly people, even those with Alzheimer's disease. Ginkgo helps maintain capillary blood circulation to the brain (supporting memory and concentration), heart, and all extremities and is available from most pharmacies, and health food stores. You need to take a minimum of 120 milligrams a day for it to be effective as a memory aid.

"The higher up you go, the more mistakes you're allowed. When at the top, if you make enough of them, it's considered your style."

FRED ASTAIRE

Defining idea…

How did it go?

Q **I have the most awful fear that I will forget someone's name as I introduce them to another person. It's happened to me a few times and it's so embarrassing. Any suggestions about how to deal with this?**

A *A name can vanish and then return just as you no longer need it. How come you can recall the name of everyone in your class at school but then forget the name of the person you have just been chatting with? I think the best way out is to make light of it as though you have had a highly unusual memory lapse; make the moment a funny one. You probably feel worse than the person whose name you have mislaid.*

Q **I was in the middle of giving an amusing speech at my daughter's wedding and I forgot the anecdote I was about to tell to make everyone fall down laughing. It was the whole point of my speech. What can I do to prevent something like that from happening again?**

A *Ouch, that can be something you want to erase from your memory, but of course you never will. The brain seems to be very selective about what it recalls and what it manages to make you forget. If there is a next time, make a few notes and keep them on hand. If you aren't an experienced speaker no one will mind if you have to refer to them now and then—and the audience will be just as nervous as you are if it goes wrong. Try to laugh it off.*

14

If I love you, will you love me back?

We all want to be loved, need to be loved, and we blossom when we are in loving company.

This seems to gather momentum when we are menopausal, when only the best kind of friendship will do.

This was very challenging to write because one minute I sounded like I was writing some sickly poem for a Valentine's card and the next as though I was trying to be some spiritual guru. Actually all I wanted to say was simple: "Love your friends as you would like them to love you."

Unconditional friendship is an approach to life, not something that can be switched on and off. If you work hard on yourself and get this right through menopause, then all the other aspects of friendship come together quite naturally. Unconditional friendship is a learning experience. If we make the conscious decision to choose it as our daily practice, our personality blooms and flourishes. We grow. So how can you experience closer friendships in menopause?

Here's an idea for you...

When you need some extra support through a crisis in your friendship and need some help to focus on what you should do next, try these essences. They give you a moment to reflect and to expand your thinking.
Pomegranate: **Regulates hormone production, increases libido, acceptance of femininity**
Morning Glory: **Eases emotional pain and stimulates the production of hormones**
Moonstone: **Addresses all female problems from pelvic disorders to ridding the body of toxins**
Pink Tourmaline: **Balances the male/female energies within the body; promotes joy and peace during periods of growth and change**

Find more possibilities at www.thenaturalsanctuary.com.

Find a time to think about where in your menopausal life you feel resentful, or have fearful feelings about where your needs around friendship are not being met. If you need help with this part then find someone who will help you feel safe and loved during the process. Talk about it honestly and ask for honest feedback. Recalling the event or person that upset you will give you a starting point.

Think about how you feel when a friend challenges you or is disrespectful in some way or other. What is your reaction now that you are menopausal? Do you immediately feel insulted or hurt? How does your reaction affect the situation for you or your friend?

Take time out to really listen and be there for your friends even if this takes the form of writing to them, calling them now and then, or seeing them once a week. Friends need to know they are cared for, and now that you are menopausal you will find some of the greatest, most rewarding friendships you have ever had. Unconditional friendship can really only happen when you feel guilt-free and switch off from all those "I should be doing something else" thoughts. Unconditional friendship is about sharing fun, being frivolous, and being indulgent.

But the most valuable thing about friendship through menopause, and the rest of your life, is that it also allows you to experience forgiveness at a very deep and profound level. One of the most challenging and most liberating things we can do in menopause is to forgive and to ask for forgiveness, whether something is our fault or not. Holding a grudge is damaging for your health, both physically and emotionally, and should no longer be part of your life in any shape or form. That's what unconditional friendship is about: It means knowing you love your friend so much that they could never hurt you. Not because you have made it clear you will ditch them if they do, but because their negative action has no impact on you. We can be restored and revitalized through offering ourselves totally to our friendships, in the knowledge that we are loved and respected or valued back.

Forgiveness is not submission—you need to travel through various painful processes before you can forgive wholly. If you approach your menopausal life from a place of unconditional love then you can achieve something: You can get in touch with others at a very deep level and also begin to get to know your own real self.

It's not just women your own age that can be good friends but also those a lot younger. See IDEA 50, *Gorgeous, sexy, and I hate you!*, for ways of making younger women your allies.

Try another idea…

"We shelter children for a time; we live side by side with men; and that is all. We owe them nothing, and are owed nothing. I think we owe our friends more, especially our female friends."

FAY WELDON

Defining idea…

61

How did it go?

Q **I simply don't have the time to spend hours working on myself—I am a mom who is menopausal. I had my son when I was 49; he's now 2. I end up giving to him all day long and have no time to give to friends anymore. What can I do?**

A *Could you still see friends who have older children and get them to help you a little? If their kids could play with your son you'd have time to talk and reconnect with your friends again. Or maybe you need to tell your friends you miss them? That might open the door for them to discover ways for you all to spend time together again.*

Q **One close friend gave me a book that recommended women going through menopause spend three days every full moon and three days every new moon doing a little ceremony to gather power. She wants me to do this with her as she feels it will bring us closer. I really don't have the time or inclination to do this but I do like my friend. What can I do?**

A *You can be direct and say a clear no. You'll probably be better off chatting together about things that matter to you both once a month than doing something one of you resents six days a month. Unconditional friendship means you can say no.*

15

Don't you just love water?

Water is the substance of life. Our planet is covered in it. Our bodies are 70 percent water. We use water to wash, bathe, and drink.

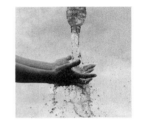

One of the greatest comforts you will discover, if you haven't already, is the vital role water will play in easing menopausal discomfort in all sorts of ways.

Even just thinking about water can change your mood instantly. Whenever I feel a weepy menopausal moment coming on I try to close my eyes and picture myself floating away on a raft sailing on a clear blue sea. I can almost hear the waves and smell the water. The world stops for a few moments and I have time to restore myself.

Menopause will be a time when you appreciate water possibly more than at any other time in your life.

Here's an idea for you... **Buy a little solar-powered fountain for your garden or balcony. There is nothing as soothing or as enchanting as sitting and watching the water falling; the sound is restful, too. These are quite cheap now and very easy to install. Solar water features require no wiring, as they gain their power from a solar panel that must be placed in the sun. They require no plumbing, either, as they simply recycle water or float on your pond.**

DRINKING IT

As you'd expect, water is the greatest hydrator there is and without water, we are dead. Drinking plenty of water is vital when you are menopausal; it will help flush away toxins, hydrate you, and keep you feeling alert and awake. Water is the single best thing there is for staying healthy. Your blood pressure, kidneys, liver, joints, and digestion all require water to function properly. In addition, water will keep your skin plumped and soft. Menopause is a time of drying out and you might want to run to alcohol, tea, coffee, or fizzy drinks for comfort, but all these are diuretics and actually make you feel worse, not better.

Drinking lots of water will keep you fit: You will not become physically tired as quickly and you will be mentally "on the ball" when your water reservoirs are filled up. Drink at least eight 8-ounce glasses of water a day, or more if you get a lot of exercise. Do not wait until you are thirsty. The very best thing is to start and finish each day with a glass of water, because while you sleep your body loses water. Finally, when the weather is hot, drink room temperature or warm water—it's absorbed much faster than iced water.

Defining idea...

"I like flowers. I also like children, but I do not chop off their heads and keep them in bowls of water around the house."

GEORGE BERNARD SHAW

VISITING IT

A day by the sea will invigorate you through menopause. It's especially effective if you can get out beyond the crowds, walk along, and breathe in the sea air and take in the sound, color, and sheer energy force the sea offers.

If you can't get to the sea, then sit by a pond or lake in a city park and just relax. Even being close to water can undo stress and make menopause a little easier to live with. Can you run out at lunchtime and get to a park for half an hour? Even a couple of times a week will help. After work, head to your local pool for a quick dip and as you swim you will ease aching joints, help erase menopausal headaches, and become more supple and aware of your body.

BATHING IN IT

Most of us find nothing nicer than a comforting, deep bath. At home, add organic oils or essences to your bathwater as well. Try sea salts and enjoy a blissful detox in your own private sea. Or use Dead Sea bathing products if you really want to tone and restore. These are marvelous tonics and bursting with minerals. I feel my bathroom is my own oasis of calm and even though I share it with other family members, my bathing and luxuriating hour is mine, and I am not to be disturbed.

Go to IDEA 3, *Use those green fingers*, for tips on how to make the best use of precious rainwater.

Try another idea...

"Be careful what you water your dreams with. Water them with worry and fear and you will produce weeds that choke the life from your dream. Water them with optimism and solutions and you will cultivate success."

LAO TZU

Defining idea...

65

How did it go?

Q **Ever since I started menopause, I have been unable to drink alcohol or coffee, as they both gave me nasty headaches. I now love drinking cool water but I live in the countryside in an old house and can't always get bottled water easily. Is tap water safe?**

A *You should always let the tap run for at least five minutes before drinking tap water, as most is contaminated with chlorine or fluoride and this allows the excess to run off. If you have old lead water pipes then get these replaced with more modern ones as the lead can leech into the water.*

Q **I would like to stop buying plastic bottles for water since they are so environmentally unfriendly but I really want to drink as much safe water as I can. What are the alternatives?**

A *You could have a home water-purifying system. You make one purchase, all your water from then on is filtered, and all the nasty stuff is taken out. You can also buy pitchers with built-in filter systems now, and we can all use conventional water filters.*

16

Only the best on my plate, please!

The demand for organic, pesticide-free food is increasing rapidly—and for good reason.

The National Cancer Institute states that 30 percent of insecticides, 60 percent of herbicides, and 90 percent of fungicides are known to cause cancer.

These chemicals can also lead to damage of both your nervous and hormonal systems. When you are menopausal and your hormonal system is already compromised, the last thing you need to do is pile on the complications through eating commercially grown food that you know is not going to do you any favors at all.

Organic fruits and vegetables are grown without the use of artificial fertilizers and heavy-duty chemical toxins; natural methods of pest and disease control are used instead. Organic produce isn't just safer, there is also little doubt that once you have tasted organic stuff it's hard to go back to the tasteless, churned-out fodder passed off for food. Food that is highly processed has lost so much of its nutritional

Here's an
idea for
you...

Eat in organic restaurants. If you are in London then try the Duke of Cambridge—a super organic pub that stocks organic beers, wines, and locally sourced organic food. Fish is from non-depleted stocks, caught using sustainable methods, and nothing the pub manager, Geetie Singh, offers is processed or packaged. Check out www.naturalmatters.net for others, or search online for places local to you.

value that it is no more than a "filler." Now that you are menopausal you don't need fillers, you need food that is going to work for you, make you feel great, and do your body and soul some good as well. Choose wisely with other things, too. Go for meat and poultry that has been allowed free-range access and fed organically; try not to buy farmed fish. Dairy foods should also be sourced from organic farms.

Although supermarkets offer a limited range of organic foods, their choice is somewhat artificial and may involve food traveling huge distances. You are better off at a farmers' market, an organic farm shop, or getting one of those organic delivery services now widely available. You might need to test these out, though, as when I had one I was left with so much food—and there wasn't room for any more soup in the freezer. Look on the Internet or read up in magazines like *Ecologist* (see www.theecologist.org), which is crammed with information about where to buy the best organic foods.

Your body is already dealing with a suspect water supply and polluted air. A wholesome organic diet is not a fad but a way of life, and once you are converted you won't ever look back. Your radiant skin, clearer eyes, enhanced taste buds, and increased energy levels will be

See IDEA 24, *How heavy are you today?*, for other ways to improve your eating habits.

Try another idea…

noticeable and your body will feel as though it is yours again once it isn't working overtime dealing with all the poisons loaded into it every day. Organic food will give you a better range of nutrients and as the practice of growing organic often involves crop rotation—just like the old days—you can be sure the soil in which the veggies have been grown is not depleted but enriched with minerals. You don't have to waste as much food either, as organic fruits and vegetables don't need peeling— simply give it a good scrub. As so much of the food's goodness lies just beneath the skin you will be retaining all the benefits.

While you are thinking organic, it is worth remembering that cleaning products ought to be organic as well. Germs in the home are not the fearsome enemies the ads on television would like us to think they are. I always used too much of the most severe cleaners and bleaches I could find, thinking I was doing a good job and keeping my home protected. However, when I read that germs get tougher and nastier over time because all these things can influence their evolution, I began to opt for safer, friendlier products. Organic foods and organic cleansers go hand in hand.

"For years I've been trying to change the fashion industry from within, with little success. A huge UK chain wouldn't publicize the collection I'd designed as organic because they were afraid people would ask what was wrong with their other clothes."

KATHARINE HAMNETT

Defining idea…

69

During menopause, I only want to eat foods grown or sourced by people who care about what I eat. I want to feel nurtured and safe with my diet. It has to be worth trying.

How did it go?

Q   I was given some wonderful flowers for my fiftieth birthday and love my house being filled with them. Then I heard that flowers could be dangerous to your health because of all the chemicals they are covered in to keep them alive. What is going on?

A   *You are quite right, there are no regulations on the use of pesticides on imported cut flowers, and these can be liberally sprayed and grown with a cocktail of chemicals, fungicides, and fumigants. As you inhale the scent from these flowers, you are absorbing these chemicals, as well as support- ing an unsavory farming method. Keep to flowers and foliage grown in your own garden or found in ethical garden centers. It is all for the good of your menopausal body and mind.*

Q   I used to love rum and Coke, but since menopause I have found I am intolerant to rum and am unsure whether it's a good idea to drink soda without the rum. Can you help?

A   *When you are menopausal and at risk of osteoporosis the last thing you need is a drink now known to contain a heady mixture of tooth- and bone-destroying acids. According to the FDA, aspartame, a sweetener used in most colas, is associated with mood swings, memory loss, headaches, joint pain, and fatigue. Aren't you possibly already battling with some of those issues as it is? Lay off the soda, diet or otherwise.*

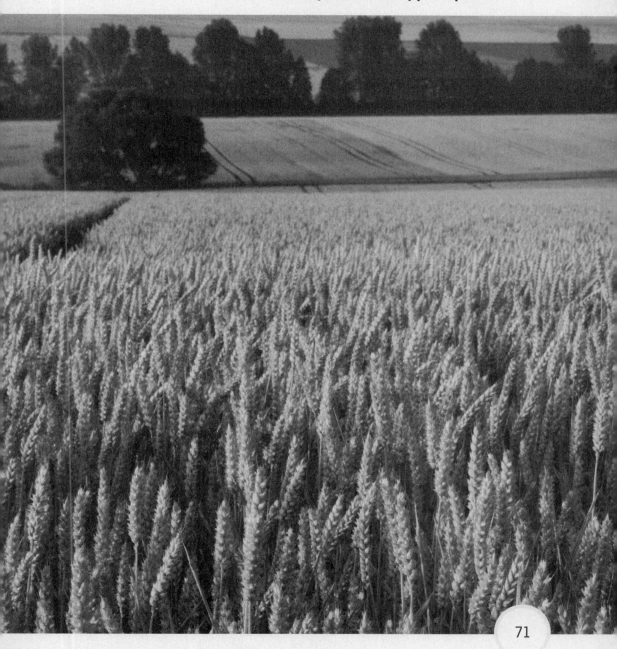

71

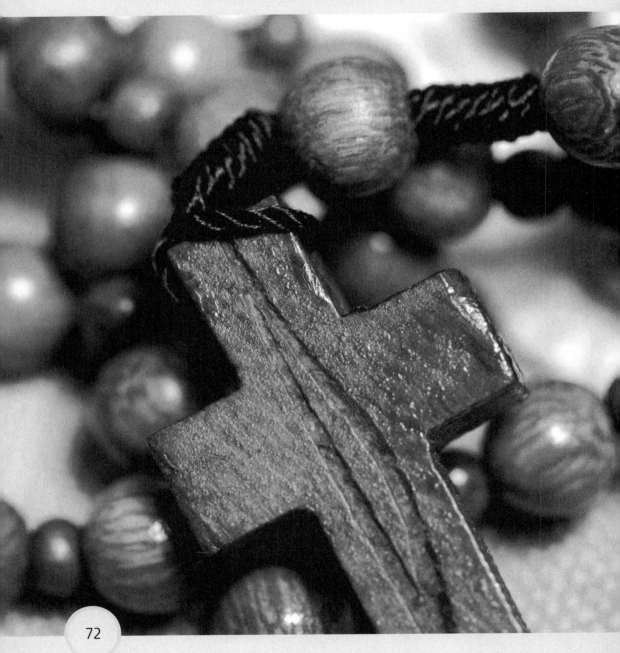

17

Now you've found religion

Churches seem to be half-empty these days and the women who do attend are, overall, of menopausal age.

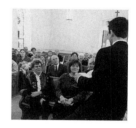

All the things about life, death, and religion you said you would think about "later" are now coming home to roost.

You can hear the little voice in the background asking, "What if it's all true after all?" and saying, "There has to be more to life than this..."

Now, if you go to church on a Sunday morning, the chances are that most of the congregation will be made up of women, and not just any women but women over the age of forty. Just listening to a hymn at a wedding or funeral can reduce the most skeptical to tears. Of course, grandchildren arriving inspire love, hope, and fear in the hearts of most women—the cycle of life repeating itself, the way your grandchild looks so like your firstborn, all reaffirm that life is precious and you want a sense of hope, renewal, and eternity.

If you are feeling hollow and want something more in your life you have a couple of options. You can go to any one of the many beautiful churches or places of worship

Here's an idea for you…

A spiritual life doesn't just mean church. You might find it useful to read books about other women and their spiritual journey through life, especially if you want more to your life than the routine you are in. Disrupt your pattern a little and see what takes its place. Let go of the everydayness and allow spontaneity in. Take an inspirational book to the bathroom with you, and as you bathe to wash away the day so you bathe to wash away your fixed ideas about your life.

and confess, beg forgiveness, promise undying devotion, and attend services regularly but not really change anything at a deep level. Alternatively, you can look inside your soul and ask yourself what exactly you are looking for. Life is not an endless round of shopping, meals, a film, and bed. Even your intellectual pursuits might not hit the spot anymore. At menopause, you know there is something else.

One woman told me that she found reading poetry a real source of personal inspiration. She read the poets she had studied at school and found she actually understood them this time around. That led her to want to read more and more until she joined a class and eventually began writing poetry herself for pleasure.

Another rediscovered her love for walking and for nature. So she decided to make changes in her personal life to the extent that she moved to a more environmentally friendly home. She became very aware of waste and of being more self-reliant. She learned how to keep chickens, grow vegetables, make her own jams and chutneys. All of the things she mocked as a businessperson suddenly began to make sense to her and she thrived through menopause because these changes satisfied her at the level of her soul.

If you want to change something, where does that change have to begin? It has to be with you. Forget all the blaming and the hunting for excuses that your partner is the reason you never "made it," or that your awful upbringing has held you back, or that the nuns at school wrecked any chance of a happy relationship… Now is the time to take stock.

IDEA 11, *Picture this…*, is about becoming aware of the power of thought and quiet.

Try another idea…

Rediscover what you love doing, from making soup to traveling to helping out at a charity event. Your own personal awakening is just waiting to be discovered. It often involves making your life simpler but more fulfilling at the same time. As soon as you find it you will know and understand your place in the world. But you can't wait for it to come to you. You have to unearth it, and make whatever you find deeply nurturing for your way of life.

"The sole purpose of human existence is to kindle a light of meaning in the darkness of mere being."

CARL JUNG

Defining idea…

How did it go?

Q   **I'm 47 and depressed, and have been so for the past couple of years. Nothing in my life has worked out the way I hoped or imagined it would and everything feels so pointless. How can I begin to get my life back?**

A   *First, you must see your doctor and check that there is nothing physically wrong with you that is causing your depression. Once you get some advice, then maybe you could search for what it is you need to make your life feel better again. A belief in yourself and what you can give to the world will set you on a positive road. Depression is often a signal that the time has come to move on and forward. There is no better way to move forward than to try to put your own feelings on hold and go out and help others in a voluntary capacity. Weird as it sounds, it really seems to work.*

Q   **I would love to meditate but find it hard to sit still for long enough. My legs begin to twitch and my mind wanders all over the place. Where am I going wrong?**

A   *We all find meditation difficult to begin with because we live at such a fast pace and it can feel wrong to simply do "nothing." But you can meditate while you are walking, watching a candle flicker, painting, or just sitting in your favorite chair. Try to close down any distractions, put on a calming tape if it helps, and let go: Simply try letting go of all the thoughts buzzing around. It takes some practice until it feels comfortable so be prepared for that. Breathe in deeply and follow your breath until you notice your body relaxing at a very deep and profound level.*

18

Ever been needled?

Acupuncture is believed to have been discovered when a man was shot through the arm with an arrow...

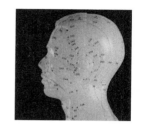

...but when a second arrow struck him, it relieved the pain from the first.

Acupuncture, a branch of traditional Chinese medicine (TCM), has been practiced in China for more than 2,000 years. This ancient medical treatment is based on regulating the body's Qi (pronounced "chee"), or "life energy," which flows in the body along pathways called meridians. Hundreds of acupuncture points can be opened, like gates, to balance and harmonize the flow of Qi, relieving pain and many other symptoms of menopause. Western acupuncture (also called medical acupuncture) is more recent and is now taught and practiced widely in the West, following a growth in popularity in the '70s.

Menopause might be a time when your body's balance of "yin" and "yang" energy is actually out of balance and acupuncturists will want to re-create a harmonious relationship between these two. Yang is warming and enlivening. When you have an ample supply of yang, you feel energetic. If your yang becomes weak, you may have a tendency to become lethargic, tired, and cold, and may have problems with your digestion, urination, or a decreased interest in sex. Women in menopause can often have weaker yin and feel very warm and dry, with hot flashes, flushed complexions, and dry lips and throats. These symptoms illustrate that when the cool yin is weakened, the warm yang becomes too prominent.

Here's an idea for you... **Acupressure works on the same points as acupuncture, but you apply pressure instead of needles. You can do it yourself, so this could become a valuable aid for easing your menopausal symptoms once you've mastered a few basic skills, and the results are usually felt fairly quickly. For instance, if you feel a menopausal sleepless night coming on, press below the knee—slightly to the right of off-center on the right leg, and slightly to the left of off-center on the left leg—and then apply pressure lightly to the center of each wrist.**

Practitioners pierce the skin using very fine sterilized needles and insert these into "acu-points" on the pathways known as meridians. Menopausal symptoms can occur when the Qi in some of the meridians becomes weak or blocked. When a needle stimulates these blockages, Qi flows through the body, clearing out energy blockages and rebalancing the body. Even though menopause is not a sign of ill health or disease, research has shown that acupuncture can be highly effective in alleviating its symptoms.

It will also allow you the time to listen to your own body and especially to the more subtle feelings you might have about any aspect of menopause. You might think a niggling ache in a joint is nothing, but your acupuncturist will want to know more about it: the intensity of sensation, when it is most acute, and when it subsides. She will check your tongue for shape, color, and coating and read your pulse on both wrists in three different positions. Once she has checked your body for any swelling, or areas that are particularly sensitive, she will want to know about your diet and any preferences for sweet, sour, or bitter foods as well as the regularity of your digestive patterns. Your sleeping habits and your body's response to temperature will also be of interest to her before she makes a diagnosis and offers you a course of treatment for menopause.

For further ways to release old patterns and feel good about yourself try IDEA 48, Sticky moments.

Try another idea…

The British Medical Association carried out a two-year study into the effectiveness of acupuncture and concluded that it should be more readily available to patients. There seems to be little doubt these days that it works and most people know someone who has tried it. You will probably need to keep up with your treatments in order to keep menopausal symptoms at bay but this will be a pleasant thing as many women report they love their treatments and find the hour with their acupuncturist highly relaxing and enjoyable. Some practitioners, though, might tend to two patients at one time and if you don't want to discuss your particular symptoms in earshot of another patient, tell your practitioner this and be treated in private—or be recommended to another acupuncturist.

"The only way to keep your health is to eat what you don't want, drink what you don't like, and do what you'd rather not."

MARK TWAIN

Defining idea…

79

How did
it go?

Q   **I am struggling with menopausal symptoms and have heard great things about acupuncture but I'm terrified of pain. Will it hurt me at all?**

A   *No. Most people enjoy treatment and find it very comfortable, restful, and relaxing. Sometimes the needle insertion feels like a quick pinch that rapidly subsides. Some people report a mild tingling, heaviness, warmth, or a dull ache at the acupuncture point, which is a sensation of Qi moving. Generally, sessions last about an hour, in which the patient rests or naps. After treatment, you can expect to feel less pain, more energy, and a heightened sense of well-being.*

Q   **I would like to try acupuncture as I have had hot flashes, night sweats, and am very irritable, but I need something that will work quickly and that won't take forever and hundreds of treatments before I feel any benefits. How many treatments am I likely to need?**

A   *The number of treatments required depends on the severity of your symptoms. For chronic menopausal conditions, a longer course of treatment is normally required than for those with less severe symptoms. Within the first four to six sessions, you and your practitioner will know how effective the treatment is and after that a clear treatment plan can be suggested.*

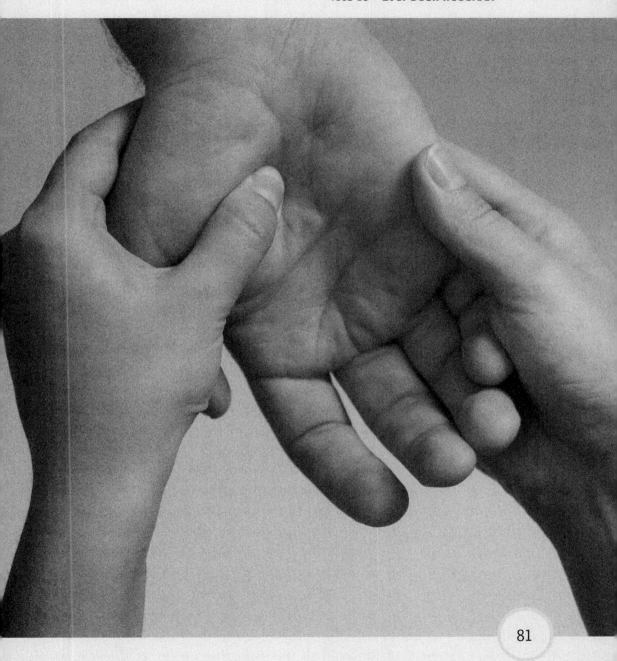

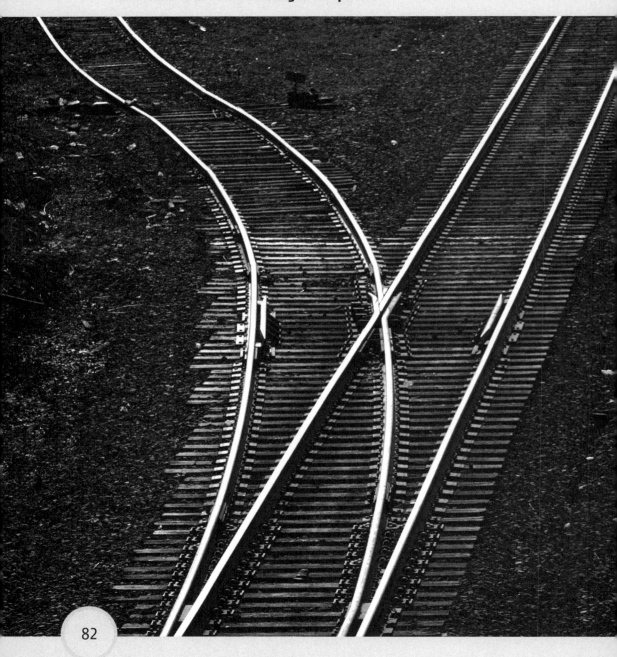

19

All change

Why not? You deserve to change everything if you so wish. Back to school? Get that promotion? Go for it, girl!

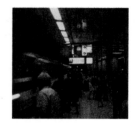

If you know intellectually and emotionally that a change or break in your career would do you a world of good, why do you keep putting it off?

A job or career that doesn't reflect your heart's desire is a ghastly a way to spend your precious time. When you are menopausal, it is even more important that you find the best possible outlet for your ideas, intelligence, and life experience.

If you have outstayed the reason why you went for your particular job in the first place, or if you stay in it for the security, the predictability, or for the "better the devil you know," your menopausal mind won't thank you. It hates what is predictable and it is desperate to get up and screech at you to go a little crazy and actually follow your heart.

Menopause is the perfect time to go for something you will find really interesting: You will be looking for a way to make your mark and this could be it. Take every-

Here's an idea for you... **If your critical voice is preventing you from making more challenging moves in your life then you will need to find ways to quiet it, especially if it starts telling you, "You'll never get that job... what will other people think... who do you think you are..." You need to find a safe way to communicate with and not simply react to your inner critic or you could make choices that are the wrong ones. Write down all your fears about moving on and then confront each item on that list. Don't let limiting beliefs stand in your way and don't fear change.**

thing into account—your finances, family, travel, and other commitments. In my experience, most women who begin something new during their menopause usually make a total success of it.

NEW GROUND

When looking for a new job, make sure you are fully up to speed on the job specs. If you feel you could give something valuable to the position you are applying for, then do not sit on your assets, but go for it. Be prepared for a tough interview by asking your partner to quiz you on every aspect of the job. On the big day, look and feel your best. Everyone applying will be nervous, as—possibly—will those giving the interview. Even the act of applying will inject excitement into your life and you will be acknowledging that you are at a very special time of your life where you want to make a valid contribution to your workplace. If you aren't offered the job, ask for an appraisal so you learn from the experience.

FURTHER EDUCATION

Universities welcome mature students with open arms; after all, you have life experience and that counts for so much in any course. Ask for a prospectus, visit a university to get the feel of it, and listen to your heart. If you feel it is right then set your application in progress. You could be picking up on a course you once began many moons ago but had to drop for some reason. You might want to study something very new but are terrified your brain will let you down and you might not be able to crank it to full speed. If you want to, you could try correspondence courses, which offer home-based, flexible study options.

If you feel nervous about being with younger people then go to IDEA 50, *Gorgeous, sexy, and I hate you!*, to help you feel more confident about communicating with a different generation.

Try another idea…

IF I SHOULD FAIL?

Promotion is a good option to challenge and stretch you mentally and physically. But if you fail to get the promotion you were after this time, so what? Don't get stuck in a menopausal gloom about it but pick yourself up and start again. If you don't get into school, ditto. The important thing is that you have started changing your life—and what can be better than that? Better to fail in a spectacular fashion and be remembered for that than for never having tried at all.

"Your work is to discover your work and then with all your heart to give yourself to it."
THE BUDDHA

Defining idea…

How did it go?

Q   **I always used to give my best at work but lately I am really concerned because I am bored stiff and can find nothing to inspire me. I do the bare minimum and I constantly clock-watch or long for weekends. I hate the fact that I am wishing my life away. How can I make a change?**

A   *Is there some skill or interest you have that you could convert into a freelance business? It sounds as though you need a brand-new working environment and a change of routine as much as needing a new challenge. It's never too late to seek advice from a career counselor.*

Q   **I feel like a hamster in a wheel as I go around and around doing the same thing day in, day out. I am not skilled and have no qualifications, so choices are strictly limited. I am in need of something to inspire and motivate me. How can I find an interesting job?**

A   *You could go to your local employment center and talk with them about a realistic appraisal of your situation. Many jobs offer on-site training and will support continuing education for you to get qualifications, no matter how old you are. Someone I know has just started a bricklaying course—at the age of 48—and she says she is the only menopausal woman she knows who is surrounded by 18-year-old guys all day long. She loves it. Think big and broad.*

20

Do you like thunder and lightning?

The questions a homeopath asks might seem very odd at first, but it's all about getting to know and understand everything about you during menopause.

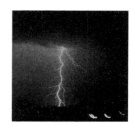

Homeopathy treats the person and not the ailment.

There are two forms of homeopathy, one ancient and another more modern, and that principle exists with both. It has been in worldwide use for more than 200 years. Samuel Hahnemann, a German doctor, organized it into a formal science in the late eighteenth and early nineteenth centuries, although the notion of "like cures like" can be traced back to Hippocrates 2,000 years ago. Its name comes from two Greek words: "homios" meaning "like" and "pathos" meaning "suffering."

Menopausal symptoms usually respond very well to homeopathy and are well worth considering as soon as your menopause begins. Visiting a homeopath can be a hugely rewarding and satisfying experience because your consultation takes in the whole of you and asks you to consider things you might think are completely irrelevant to menopause, such as whether or not you like thunder.

As quite a speedy person, I was agitated at first at the slow and deliberate questioning the homeopath employed as she looked at me. I could not see the point of another crazy question but when she asked me whether I liked windy weather, something in me clicked and I could see where she was coming from. Everything she asked I either hated or loved. She was identifying me and how I felt. Her questions were all part of her figuring out why I was suffering from blinding menopausal headaches. Each consultation is unique. Everything about you—your physical, mental, and emotional state—is taken into consideration.

Your personality will play a big part in assessing where menopause might be throwing up challenges for you, and even your face and other physical features will determine the treatment. Be prepared to be asked about your lifestyle, any patterns of disease within your family, and your relationships. Try to be as open and as honest as you can; the only judgment your homeopath is making about you is what treatment to give you. I know one woman who was embarrassed when she was asked about her relationship so she told a lie in answer. That led to another lie and in the end she said she felt she had almost become another person and was in a panic that an incorrect treatment might be administered. She had to go back over all her comments. Even then, it was all right: the homeopath asked whether she often felt she was being judged and had to tell untruths. Her fibs and then confession, far from being a diversion, actually helped the homeopath figure out

Here's an idea for you…

If you need fast relief and cannot get to a homeopath immediately, you could visit your nearest pharmacy or health store and go to their homeopathic treatment section. Here you will generally find an easy-to-understand chart explaining which treatment to take for what, and there may be an assistant on hand to help you choose. Although these treatments are more general, they will stand you in good stead until you can make an appointment with a practitioner.

what was going on with her and how to help her menopause.

If you try homeopathy you won't have to worry about any harmful effects, as there aren't any. The treatments don't have any chemical action but work by stimulating your own defense mechanism and healing system. The results of good homeopathic treatment can go beyond just treating your menopause but, like all good therapies, can have a lasting and permanent influence on your life and well-being.

One of the great things reported about homeopathy and menopausal women is that it will improve your mental outlook on life and increase your energy levels as well as deal with the more physical problems that have been bothering you since your menopause began.

Homeopathy's aim is to offer you a rapid and permanent cure for any and all of your menopausal symptoms. You probably already assume that you have to put up with a certain amount of discomfort but a homeopath would claim this does not necessarily have to be the case at all. Your homeopath will find a treatment aimed at really getting to the bottom of and curing your menopausal ailments rather than just relieving them.

Homeopathy gets to the very root of who you are, so why don't you do the same with your home and get back to having a clear vision about how you want to live? See IDEA 21, *Space Clearing*, for thoughts about what to do.

Try another idea...

"Homeopathy is the safest and more reliable approach to ailments and has withstood the assaults of established medical practice for over 100 years."

YEHUDI MENUHIN

Defining idea...

89

How did it go?

Q **I would like to visit a homeopath but am not sure if it might be a waste of money as I am taking drugs for a minor heart complaint. Will a homeopath treat me even though I am on prescribed drugs?**

A *Homeopathic remedies can be used alongside conventional drugs. Treatment can help reduce or even remove the need for many drugs, but this must be done gradually under the supervision of your doctor.*

Q **My friend told me homeopathy was exposed as useless in a recent report and I shouldn't go near it but my menopausal hot sweats are driving me to distraction. Is it safe?**

A *Homeopathy is a complete system of medicine and is the second most widely used form of medicine for primary care in the world today. Roughly 9 percent of the population in the UK are regular users, for example, and its popularity is rising again in spite of damning reports. Homeopathy should work very well with easing your hot sweats and should provide you with other benefits. If you're worried you have a serious medical problem you should consult your doctor, too.*

21

Space Clearing

Space Clearing may sound a little hippie and New Age, so why do it? Isn't a good, old-fashioned spring cleaning of your house enough?

Does it mean you have to throw away your favorite knickknacks, ornaments, and all those funny pictures the kids did when they were little?

No! Space Clearing for menopause is about channeling all that newfound creativity and energy that you've discovered during this special time of your life. Space Clearing is an ancient art—used by Native Americans, the Celts, and the Mayan civilizations, for example—but it's also about cleansing your home, your personal space, and focusing your energies in ways that allow you to rid yourself of the stresses and anxieties of menopause. It is a positive act, an affirmation of your self and your home, through which you will find inner peace and harmony. Space Clearing is a way in which you make a bold statement about the type of woman you are. Menopause is a new beginning, the start of a fresh phase in your life.

Here's an idea for you... **When you see a menopausal friend struggling with the clutter she might live in, have a chat with her and insist on helping her clear her home up. Do it well and give it as a birthday gift or in exchange for something she might offer you.**

So, if Space Clearing is more than polishing and cleaning, then how is it done? Well, here are some very simple ideas to guide you:

- **S**tart with looking at your home. Walk calmly from room to room without any interruptions from others, so take the phone off the hook, turn off the TV or the radio.
- **P**repare yourself. Take a bath with your favorite scent in it; eat a light, nourishing meal first. Begin with a clear head and if you want others to help you, make sure they will be respectful of what you are doing, that they know how important this is to you.
- **A**ssess the way your home is now. Try to be objective about all the things you have accumulated and the layout of each room.
- **C**hoose the right day. A clear bright one is best. Begin by thinking about it a few days before… you'll find yourself looking forward to this special day!
- **E**qually important is what you wear when you look around. Wear comfortable clothes and take off your slippers or shoes. This will let you connect with your surroundings in a physical and spiritual way.

- Concentrate on what you are doing. Look at all your furniture and how it is placed. Look at everything that's around you and think about its own very special meaning.

While you're clearing out the outside, why not give your inside attention as well? See IDEA 26, *Cranky colonics*, for more info.

Try another idea...

- Let your creativity loose! Allow yourself to think about any changes you may want to make, trust yourself, and really believe in the freedom of your gut instincts.
- Examine each room slowly and thoughtfully. Begin at the front door and, breathing deeply and walking with purpose, imagine you are surrounded by light and energy.
- Ask yourself what you really need around you, how much of your living space is cluttered? Can you move freely from one space to the next? How does your home "flow"?
- Recycle. Know that those ornaments, pictures, clothes—all of those things that you don't really need—will benefit others if you take them to a secondhand shop.
- Imagine yourself in harmony with the physical and spiritual world. This will guide you through making some difficult decisions, as well as simultaneously finding new levels of energy and an inner balance.
- Necessary requirements are looking in corners, under beds, or behind the sofa. You'll need to clear out all those dark and hidden spaces that nobody sees, but which you know are there.
- Gather your family together after you have traveled around your home. Explain to them what you are doing and why. Let them know that these profound changes are being made to create a harmonious space for the benefit of all.

"The space needs to be occupied after the ceremony—meaning you should not go away for the weekend just after the ceremony, etc.—you do want to bask in the new, clean energy and consciously feel the new path set in motion."

MARGIT, Canada's first Space Clearing practitioner

Defining idea...

Paying attention to your home in this way not only frees you from the negative thoughts, feelings, and emotions you may have about menopause, but will help to realign your energy.

When you have undergone Space Clearing, spray each room with a pleasing air freshener. Light a scented candle in the evening to enhance your mood. Your home will become a place of inspiration and fresh new ideas, a serene place to counteract the changes your body is experiencing.

How did it go?

Q **I have an old dinner service on display. I don't like it, but it belonged to my mother-in-law—I can't throw it away! What can I do with it?**

A *Your possessions take up your time and energy; they need cleaning and taking care of. This means they are a distraction from things you really want to do. Wrap it up carefully, box it, and put it in the attic.*

Q **I've got some ornaments I've had for years, but now I want the space again. I'm finding it hard to get rid of them. Can I give my grown-up kids things they gave me when they were young?**

A *It is hard to let things go when there's sentiment attached but explain that you'll keep the ones you really like and yes, why not offer the ornaments to them? They won't be offended, I'm sure. If they don't want them, donate them to charity and somebody will be thrilled to have them.*

22

Powerful tools, words

And isn't it incredible just how strong these little ancient shapes are and how much they can sting?

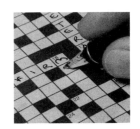

In Central America, the Mayans used words of power to influence the weather, banish illness, and to ask the favor of the gods...

The shamans of Africa are especially adept at the use of songs, chants, and words of power in the formation of a powerful form of medicine. Explorers in the Congo have documented cases in which they have seen this medicine heal the sick, bring on rainstorms, ease the pain of childbirth, and even calm the fury of raging animals—all with the utterance of a single word or phrase.

How you use words during menopause is going to have a real impact on the way you feel about yourself. Why is menopause the time to get your language right? Well, because menopause is riddled with the same old messages about feeling old, being past it, looking awful... Very few words describe it as being a welcome stage or a transition. That's why it's vital you get it right and use the appropriate positive words to describe the fact that although what you are going through is challenging, it has helped you grow.

Here's an idea for you...

If you want to lighten up a bit then buy one of those digital radios with an earphone attachment! When you can't sleep you could use the earphones and tune in to a radio station that broadcasts old comedy favorites. It's a lovely way to spend a couple of hours and will mean you don't disturb anyone—and you'll fall asleep feeling happy if you hit on the right program.

People make huge judgments about others based on how and what they have said. During menopause, when you might be feeling at odds with the world, it is painfully easy to not want to be heard. You feel out of sorts and sometimes find it hard to string two words together.

Adopt a more powerful vocabulary by:

- Stopping the negative words in your brain now.
- Replacing them with life-affirming, positive words—even if it's the last thing you feel like doing. Just do it.
- Building your own positive word dictionary full of antidotes to the words that keep you from enjoying your life.

When I am down I no longer let my menopausal "yakkety-yak" voice go on and on inside my head. I quiet it. I make the inner nagging critic go away and I replace its message with something better. I don't need to beat myself up about being menopausal every day. I tell myself that I am learning from this stage in my life, that I will make mistakes and learn from them. I am trying to live the best life I can and I will upset people sometimes, but I take responsibility for my life and I can begin again today.

But how do you start this process?

I do it through changing the words I tell myself, and through the words I now use when I speak to other people. If people are being critical or nasty about me then I don't want their words to have so much power over me that I am left paralyzed, or react with a torrent of abusive words back. So I listen first and know when to speak and when to keep quiet. Menopause certainly makes you extra-sensitive to words and this is really useful as it means you begin to use them with greater care.

Go to IDEA 36, *Musical madness*, for ways to improve the quality of your speech and to strengthen and increase your vocal cords.

Try another idea...

Someone recently told me that as we have two ears and one mouth, we are probably meant to listen more and to speak less. What she was saying was this: When you do speak, make it count.

Your menopausal mind is whirring with new ideas about your future, your present, and your past. You might be feeling downright miserable or weepy, and if you speak in a negative, downbeat way, you'll begin to feel more miserable, you'll cry more, and you'll feel alienated. It's better, far better, to stop this cycle before it becomes ingrained. Healthy thoughts and healthy words go hand in hand.

"A word after a word after a word is power."
MARGARET ATWOOD

Defining idea...

97

How did
it go?

Q **I know it's not just menopause that is making me feel depressed, but I can't find the words to tell anyone how I am feeling. I really need to get it out, but I know the words in my head don't make sense as soon as they are spoken. I feel I am quietly going crazy. What can I do to make sense of my feelings?**

A *Since you are having problems talking about what is going on, why don't you write it all down? Write as much detail as you can and keep adding to it when you feel another idea coming along. When you read over what you have written it should give you a clearer picture of what is causing the depression. Tune into what is happening to you and then you will be able to take the next step and talk it through with someone.*

Q **Since menopause started, I dread the phone at home. I work in a busy office, talk all day, and loathe the phone ringing at night, even if it's my friends. Other than turning it off, what can I do?**

A *Probably every menopausal woman reading this will know what you mean. You want to stay in touch with friends but talking on the phone after a day at work is too much. Could you leave a simple friendly message on your landline's answering machine asking them to leave you a text message on your cell phone? That way you have communicated with them and saved your sanity.*

23

Be healthy and hearty

Did you know that heart disease is the leading cause of death for women in the United States?

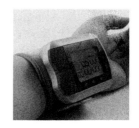

But did you know it is one of the most preventable diseases as well? Well, it is. Knowing that makes you feel a whole lot better right away.

I hate thinking I might have a potential time bomb in my chest. Both my parents died of heart disease so I know I have to look after my old ticker as well as watch out for all the signs leading up to heart disease. Mom was 60 when she died and had taken HRT since she started menopause and so thought she was protected from heart problems, as was the popular belief not too long ago. She wanted extra protection because her mom had also died of heart disease—at 60. The thing is that both my gran and mom were slim, healthy, and into whole food and organic food, ahead of their time in a way. So I know it's not just diet but a whole load of other factors that will keep me safe from heart disease.

The typical time for a woman to have a heart attack is about ten years after menopause, and then the chances are that it happens, as in the case of my mom and gran,

Here's an
idea for
you…

Check out your earlobes. They are usually bursting with blood but if they are creased then it can show a decreased blood supply through your heart—something recently discovered in the West but known by Eastern medicine for hundreds of years.

very quickly. A doctor at the hospital my mom was in told me that women tend to come for diagnosis or treatment too late, and she thought this was because women as a whole tend to take care of everyone but themselves.

So what can you do to head off heart disease? Well, you already know that it's 100 percent vital that you stop smoking. The complications of smoking-related diseases are already well documented but especially during menopause—when everything seems to be on heightened awareness—you will be more susceptible to heart disease if you haven't packed it in by now. In 2000 over five million people worldwide died as a direct result of smoking tobacco. I don't think it's worth that risk, and any woman I know who smokes now gets a lecture from me asking them to quit—today.

It's highly recommended that menopausal women have a blood-pressure check and cholesterol check at least once a year, moreso if (like me) you think there might be a problem. See your doctor and talk things through. You might feel you are wasting the doctor's time but you aren't. It's no good saying, "If only I'd gone to the doctor" once you're dead and buried, is it? Go now and get used to it.

You can also be proactive in the following ways and head off a heart crisis:

- Limit fat intake and opt for a Mediterranean diet. People in Southern Italy, Sicily, and Crete suffer fewer heart diseases than people elsewhere and they eat a diet rich in delicious foods such as vegetables, fruit, fish, a little meat, whole grain breads, and cereals. If you limit your alcohol intake to a glass a day and eat some olives you are on your way to helping your heart as well as the rest of you throughout menopause. A good diet rich in the essential fatty acids will help stave off cancer and osteoporosis as well. Eating oily fish at least three times a week will help lower your cholesterol levels, thin your blood, and therefore reduce the chances of narrowing of the arteries.

Unwind and have a good night's sleep to help keep you stress-free and take care of your heart. See IDEA 44, *Get a little shut-eye*, for ways of achieving this.

Try another idea…

- Exercise through menopause is another must. A sedentary lifestyle could make you a prime target and you need to be physically active regularly, and by that I mean taking a good brisk walk at least three to five times a week. We're talking a walk that means you feel it—about 45 minutes in duration. You can increase this as you become fitter.
- Take a vitamin E supplement as soon as your menopause begins. Research at Cambridge University and at Papworth Hospital in the UK has found that a daily dose of vitamin E can reduce the chance of having a heart attack by up to 75 percent.
- Stress factors. Now that you are menopausal you need to take time to deal with anything that is troubling you and resolve all those issues. Be proactive and creative in the ways you can deal with challenges. It's when you go over and over the same old thing without doing anything about it that the stress builds and builds. Nothing is insurmountable.

"A cheerful heart is good medicine."
THE BIBLE, Proverbs 17:22

Defining idea…

- Check out your legs for varicose veins as they, too, can be a sign that not all is well—and if there is the chance of a blood clot forming you need to get it taken care of.

How did it go?

Q **I eat well now that I'm in menopause but I love salt. Is it so dangerous?**

A   *You are better off limiting your salt intake as salt can lead to high blood pressure and this causes heart disease. It won't take long for you to get used to food without salt, especially if you substitute the taste with other foods from the sharp-tasting group, like lemons and limes squeezed over vegetables and fish.*

Q **Since I started menopause I notice that I have palpitations whenever I drink more than one cup of coffee. Is this dangerous?**

A   *Coffee gives you a buzz and makes you feel alert and awake but this can make your heart work overtime and increase palpitations. Find a coffee substitute or drink decaffeinated coffee.*

24

How heavy are you today?

Don't you think it's a little strange how one night you can go to bed feeling skinny and wake up feeling fat? What happened overnight?

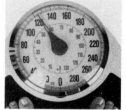

As many of us enter menopause, we might find ourselves experiencing unexplained weight gain—especially around the waist and hips—despite our best attempts to diet.

Often the methods of weight management that have worked for years are suddenly ineffective. In fact, weight gain in the abdomen is one of the most common complaints of menopausal women. It's a bit much to be told that extra weight is simply a rite of passage at this time of our lives and that we should simply accept "middle-age spread." But we don't have to. There is no reason why you should settle for anything at this stage of your life, let alone weight gain. Hormonal fluctuations at this time can result in some extra weight. But it doesn't mean you're stuck with it.

Weight loss is not about willpower or dieting. Fad diets simply don't work—over 95 percent of dieters put back on the weight they lose and more—because they oversimplify a very complicated process. We spend a fortune on diet aids that are a waste of money. Weight gain is just another symptom of a system being out of balance. To restore balance, you need to figure out what is going on at the core of your physiology and emotions.

For years, many women followed the conventional low-fat, high-carbohydrate diet, with lots of processed foods (white breads, white pasta, and other refined foods; most snacks, beer, and wine). Over time this diet can create a condition where your body converts every calorie it can into fat, even if you're dieting. The result is that while you are gaining weight, your cells are actually starving.

There is also a link between stress and body fat. Stress hormones block weight loss. This is sometimes called the "famine effect": despite adequate food, the body interprets prolonged stress as a famine, and actually stores fat thinking it's doing you a favor. Unresolved emotional issues are often the root cause of unhealthy eating habits—and once you begin to figure out your life your eating habits often get fixed as well.

"I want to be thin" is a common lament. Well, you don't have to be thin during menopause and you will certainly not do yourself any favors by being too thin or constantly trying to achieve something that is no longer possible. Your body fat serves as a little harbor for estrogen and this helps protect your heart, and also protects you from osteoporosis. You should ideally stay in your "comfortable" zone and you know where that is—probably no more

Here's an idea for you...

Increase your fiber intake. Soluble fiber, found in fruits, beans, and oats, helps control cholesterol levels because it binds with some of the cholesterol and fats in the food you eat. Insoluble fiber found in vegetables and whole grains takes anything your body doesn't need out of your system. Both are important through menopause.

than a few pounds more than you weighed before menopause. As soon as a fat day comes along, check out what emotional disturbances have played havoc with your eating.

If you want to clean up you could go for a colonic irrigation and see how you like it. See IDEA 26, *Cranky colonics*, for information about what to expect.

Try another idea...

Eating little and often is the best way when you are menopausal, as you avoid the sugar crash and won't feel weighed down with a heavy meal to digest. Little and often prevents overeating because you never feel hungry. It also keeps you alert and in a better frame of mind; this in itself will help you deal with menopausal symptoms.

Eating the right foods for you and avoiding sugary snacks will keep you fit and well fed. Food needs to nourish you, not just fill you up, and so make sure your diet contains at least the recommended five portions of fruits and vegetables every day as well as a regular intake of oily fish and some organic meats. You also need nuts, seeds, and oils for a good supply of omega-3 essential fatty acids.

Go organic wherever possible as this will limit the amount of chemicals and pesticides your body absorbs, and your body has enough to deal with through everyday living as it is. Toxins accumulate in your fat cells—and these can be hard to shift as well—so keep as clean a system as you can.

"She fitted into my biggest armchair as if it had been built round her by someone who knew they were wearing armchairs tight around the hips that season."
P. G. WODEHOUSE

Defining idea...

How did it go?

Q Now that I am menopausal should I buy those low-fat foods and prepared meals you see in supermarkets?

A *If you do go on a fat-free diet or even cut down too drastically on your "good" fats you will notice a deterioration in the condition of your skin, suffer from joint aches and pains, and could lose more of your natural vaginal lubricant. Although these are fine now and then, it is far better to prepare your own wholesome meals, balancing the fats and food yourself.*

Q I'd like to become a vegetarian since I feel I can no longer digest meat so easily. Is this safe or is my system regulated to eat meat because I've done so since I was a child?

A *It's always good to stand back and check out what you are eating and why. If you slowly substitute tofu or other soy-based foods for meat you will be keeping your diet healthy. Your body can certainly cope without meat and your digestion will probably improve no end. You may need to take zinc or iron supplements to ease you through this change of diet, and you should also consider vitamin B_{12}. Speak to your doctor or to a qualified nutritionist or dietician.*

25

"Wow! You look great!"

Now that we are menopausal should we change the way we use makeup? Most experts would say yes...

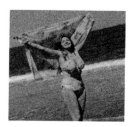

I'm not convinced, though. However, what we can review is the stage before we apply makeup. So how do we get the basics right?

According to all those beauty makeover shows we ought to trash our makeup and start again. Well, that's OK if you have a beautician on hand to pamper and make you up every time you leave the house but I imagine that if you are like me, it's not on your agenda to reconsider your makeup routine: I've spent years looking for the ultimate red lipstick and I'm not going to give up the search now that I am menopausal.

What I will reconsider, though, are things like paying more attention to my eyebrows. Until I had them reshaped professionally recently I had forgotten what a difference a neat brow can make. I can't say it was pain-free—in fact, the poor woman doing my brows had to pin me down I was yelling so loudly—but it was worth the pain. A well-shaped brow can lift and open your eyes, making you look sophisticated and more confident. Although I don't think you have to make the main objective of applying makeup, or any beauty routine, "looking younger," I do think a neat brow can knock a few years off your age and give you a boost when you are menopausal.

If your brows are truly unruly, then get them done by a professional and try to be diligent about removing any new hairs to maintain the shape. To reshape your brows yourself you'll need about forty minutes. Don't rush. Once you pluck a hair, it takes a long time to grow back. Here are the tools you'll need:

- A large mirror near a window so you can use natural light
- A good pair of tweezers
- Grooming scissors
- A small brush—an old mascara wand that's been cleaned will do

Here's an idea for you... **If you need new basics go to a beauty counter in a larger pharmacy or department store and ask them to show you what to do. They are usually really friendly and offer all sorts of tips. I usually go for a makeover when I have anything special that evening. It's free and relaxing and these women know what they are doing.**

Remember, less is more. You can always go back and pluck again. Before you pluck, determine what your best shape is. In many cases, nature has already given you an arch that will become more obvious when you remove hairs along the bottom of the brow. Don't try to copy someone else's brow—work with your own natural bone structure. Don't over-pluck or the effect can be one of making you look very serious; when you are in menopause you might want a more relaxed look. If you have been too enthusiastic, use some brownish eye shadow and then brush the hair back into place. Fill in any bald spots if necessary.

See IDEA 46, *Excuse me, can you see me?*, for other ways to increase self-esteem.

Try another idea...

Before applying eyeshadow, put a little of your foundation across your eyelid and blend it gently up toward the eyebrow. If you've got those late-night menopausal dark circles under your eyes, pop a little concealer there as well, but be sure to blend carefully. This will hide any discoloration and help set the color you're going to apply.

Once you've done your color, go for an eyelash curler; you might have had one when you were a teenager and already know the difference they can make. Through your menopause you'll probably have thinner eyelashes than before and these curlers do make the most of what you have. But choose a good one, one that will give a natural curl without yanking your lashes out, as they take a long time to grow back.

Be careful with your mascara as well, because if you are using one claiming to thicken, lengthen, or curl your lashes, it's making a lot of fibers cling to them. These mascaras can be prone to making very heavy, lumpy lashes, which can make you look tired and aged—and that's already too easy when you're menopausal as it is. Opt instead for a lighter mascara that separates and curls each lash, and use it sparingly.

"Cosmetics are a boon to every woman, but a girl's best beauty aid is still a near-sighted man."

YOKO ONO

Defining idea...

109

How did it go?

Q **I'm a 58-year-old woman with very dry skin and my makeup just doesn't go on smoothly. Is there anything you can suggest to help me?**

A *Begin by moisturizing and invest in a high-quality intensive moisturizer that will work to treat and repair skin cells. Apply your moisturizer immediately after cleansing your skin, while it is still damp. Next, always apply sunscreen with an SPF (sun protection factor) of at least 15 when headed outdoors. Use makeup created specifically for very dry skin. You can choose from creamy foundations, shadows, and blushers, as these non-powder formulas will work best for you. Not only are they incredibly easy to apply (you can actually do everything with your fingers), but they also give you the option of easily mixing in extra moisturizer if needed.*

Q **I have more wrinkles beneath my eyes than ever. This makes applying foundation difficult, as it seems to cling to the wrinkles and highlight them. What do you suggest?**

A *There are a few products you can use to minimize the appearance of wrinkles that you apply before foundation. Check out others on good cosmetics counters or at www.sephora.com.*

26

Cranky colonics

It is time to get clean inside and out. Cleanliness, as they say, is next to godliness.

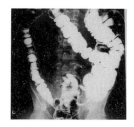

You wouldn't live in a house that hadn't been cleaned for 45 or more years, so why be one?

The liver and intestines work hard at dealing with all the crap and garbage we throw at them. They could probably do with a helping hand now and then if they are to retain their efficiency.

You might have wondered who in their right mind would dream of having a colonic irrigation. When I first heard of them, I dismissed them as being a bit on the wacko side and something I would not seriously consider. Then a colonic therapist came to stay with us a few days a week. She was my age, menopausal, and had the clearest skin I had ever seen. She was in shape and kept to a diet so perfectly you knew she would go straight to heaven.

When she asked me if I wanted a colonic, I laughed and said I did not want her poking around my rear end and then coming back to the house for supper. But she

Here's an idea for you... If you're on HRT, think about the way you take it. Try patches or creams instead of pills, as pills are absorbed from the intestines and passed immediately through the liver. A large portion of the hormone may be broken down here before it can get into general circulation, and in some people this might render the HRT ineffective or cause the liver to become overworked. Discuss it with your doctor.

insisted it was nothing like that and said it would help me with my weight, my concentration, any congestion I had, any bloating, and would make my menopause easier. As I was at the onset of menopause, I decided to go with the flow.

SKIP THIS PART IF YOU ARE SQUEAMISH!

I went to her clinic and undressed down to a towel. I then had to lie on one side while she examined my rectum for signs of disease or growths. All was clear there and so she began the process of inserting a tube with a nozzle the size of a tampon into my rectum and filling my rear end with warm water. How did it feel? Odd. I felt a weird sense of wanting to push but, of course, I couldn't. Every so often, she would stop the flow, massage my tummy, and then a valve would release the debris that was being dislodged from the intestinal walls. If you are so inclined, you can see what comes out, as the tubes are clear plastic. I am very nosy and watched with fascination as some of the previous Sunday's lunch came out almost undigested. "That's awful!" I shrieked.

She agreed and said that this type of congestion would make menopause more difficult—that toxins needed to be kept flowing out of the body. People joke that spicy food does the same thing but it doesn't at all. All that happens is the tummy is irritated and gets rid of the food fast. It doesn't sweep out the entire length of the intestines as a colonic does. Afterward, I felt slimmer, calmer, and my menopausal bloating had vanished.

See IDEA 16, *Only the best on my plate, please!*, for other ways of keeping yourself spanking clean inside and out.

Try another idea...

It is a recognized fact that colon health degrades with age—therefore it is desirable to gently and naturally detoxify and cleanse your colon regularly. As your colon is responsible for eliminating all waste from your body, it is critical to maintain a healthy colon in order to enhance your health and vitality. In a clean colon, elimination occurs on a regular basis. When your colon becomes impacted or full of material, elimination becomes infrequent and your body will process fewer vitamins and minerals from your food. I realized it was no use forking out a fortune for supplements to help with menopause if I wasn't assimilating them properly.

"Sex is interesting but it's not totally important. I mean it's not even as important (physically) as excretion. A man can go seventy years without a piece of ass, but he can die in a week without a bowel movement."

CHARLES BUKOWSKI, author

Defining idea...

I also found out about the liver, another of our waste-disposal mechanisms, and wanted to know how to help it clean out the old toxins and especially old hormones. The best thing by far for the liver is a detox routine for a few days. This one can be found in Marilyn Glenville's book *The New Alternatives to HRT*:

- Days 1–3, cut out all tea, coffee, and alcohol
- Days 3–7, drink this before you do anything else:
  - 3/4 cup lemon juice, freshly squeezed
  - 3/4 cup springwater
  - 1 clove garlic
  - 1 tablespoon organic olive oil
  - 1/2 inch ginger root, chopped
  - Mix everything in the blender and drink. Fifteen minutes later drink a cup of peppermint tea. Eat plenty of fruit and vegetables for the rest of the days that you follow this gentle regime. It will clear you out and clean you up.

Q   I am bloated. I certainly don't want a pipe shoved up my rear end but feel I could do with something to help me restore equilib- rium with my gut. What do you think would work best for me?

How did it go?

A   *You could try some other therapies to assist in a cleanse. There are probio- tics you can take that help the gut keep a healthy flora—especially useful if you have had a course of antibiotics. Give those a try.*

Q   Aren't enemas and colonics just part of a New Age fad?

A   *Not at all. The first recorded enema goes back to 1500 BC and was in Egypt where the Pharaoh had his own "guardian of the anus," a doctor employed to administer the royal colonic. In pre-revolutionary France a post-dinner enema was de rigueur and it is said Louis XIV had more than 2,000 in his lifetime. He was known for his wonderful complexion—so they could be a useful part of any menopausal management regimen.*

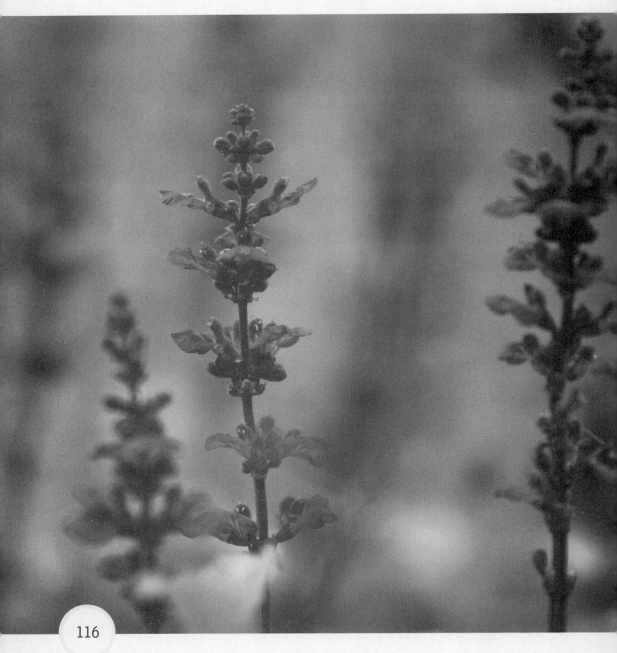

27

It's going on right under your nose

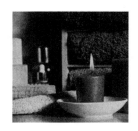

Did you know that some of the earliest documented forms of aromatherapy were found in ancient Egypt?

Some 3,000-year-old papyruses have been discovered containing remedies for all sorts of ailments, and some are identical to those used by aromatherapists today.

The modern term "aromatherapy" was coined in 1928 by the French chemist Rene-Maurice Gattefosse but combinations of oils, resins, and fragrant plants were used in some form—for ceremonial, medicinal, or pleasurable reasons—in most ancient civilizations. The ancient Egyptians used aromatic plants and their essential oils to create massage oils, medicines, embalming preparations, skin-care products, fragrant perfumes, and cosmetics. There are written accounts of aromatic oil use in China, Greece, and Babylon. In fact, the *Chinese Yellow Emperor Book of Internal Medicine*, written in 2697 BC, is the oldest surviving medical book in China: It contains information on more than three hundred plants and their properties.

Here's an idea for you...

Why not create your own dry-skin treatment for your body? Blend together one drop each of rose, patchouli, geranium, frankincense, and sandalwood oils and mix these with 2 tablespoons of evening primrose oil. Smooth this over your body after bathing and you will not only feel uplifted, but will sleep better and you will wake up with the scent still lingering in your bedroom.

Defining idea...

"Smells are surer than sights to make the heartstrings crack."

RUDYARD KIPLING

Research has shown that smelling aromatherapy oils through menopause can offer certain therapeutic benefits. Smell is the most primitive of our senses and is the only one we have directly connected to our brain.

When you inhale essential oils, they affect your brain in several ways. The essential oil compound sends a message directly to your brain—or more particularly to the part linked to memory, learning, and emotion. This can trigger change, which stimulates actual physiological responses in your body via your nervous, endocrine, or immune systems. Aromatherapy has special healing influences over menopausal problems because smell works directly on the part of the brain governing your pituitary gland, and this one governs your hormones. So, if menopause is troubling you with headaches, feelings of irritability, or mood swings, then this is a wonderful treatment to restore calm and ease your discomfort. The benefits are accumulative, so the more you take in these oils the faster your brain responds to them. Not only can you be massaged with the oils but you can have them working away in the background in your home.

When you make an appointment to see an aromatherapist about menopause, she will ask you about your medical history, your relation-ships, and any other issues you might be grappling with at the moment. Then she will ask you to undress and offer you a towel that she will expertly place to cover you up. These towels are usually warm and very comforting. She will then massage you with the appropriate oil for anything up to an hour. This massage is highly relaxing and, coupled with the smell of the oil, will release tension and produce feelings of well-being and health. The most suitable oils for menopause generally are geranium, chamomile, rose, neroli, ylang ylang, jasmine, lavender, and sage.

Bath therapy with essential oils can have profound effects, nourishing dry menopausal skin as well as reducing levels of stress and increasing and supporting blood and lymph circulation. Dosage is recommended at five to ten drops in a full bath, and the water should

IDEA 6, *Give yourself a good going-over*, will teach you other ways to create harmony in your body.

Try another idea…

"Nothing can cure the soul but the senses just as nothing can cure the senses but the soul."
OSCAR WILDE

Defining idea…

119

be warm but not hot. The essential oils should be added to the bath either once you are in it or just before you get in. Always swish the water around in order to disperse the oils in the water.

Essential oils float on the bathwater and may leave a thin film of undiluted oil on your skin in certain areas when leaving the bath. Therefore oils that are potentially irritating or sensitizing may cause reactions in people with sensitive skins.

Safety note: If any irritation occurs on your skin while bathing it may be that too much essential oil was added to the bath. Should irritation occur, rinse the area with cool water and apply a light cream without essential oils; the irritation should dissipate within an hour.

Although aromatherapy seems too good to be true, many conventional practition-ers are turning to or employing aromatherapy to complement their own form of medicine. Aromatherapy is well worth seeking out through menopause.

Q   **I love nice smells and my daughter wants to treat me to a set of oils for my home. I don't want her to waste her money. Is there a difference between fragrances and essential oils?**

How did it go?

A   *Aromatherapy oils must contain pure essential oils from plants and must not contain any added natural or synthetic substances. Pure essential oils must also appear in quantities considered to be therapeutic.*

Q   **I have been having terrible trouble sleeping since I began meno- pause a few months ago and am desperate to find something to help me unwind as well as sleep. Will aromatherapy help me get a good night's sleep?**

A   *It could be the answer you are looking for. If you put a few drops of laven- der, vetivert, and chamomile in a bowl of hot water by your bed the smells will waft around you through the night, helping you sleep like a baby. Alternatively, you could buy an aroma bowl and warming dish, a little dish you plug in and that releases the right amount of oils all throughout the night.*

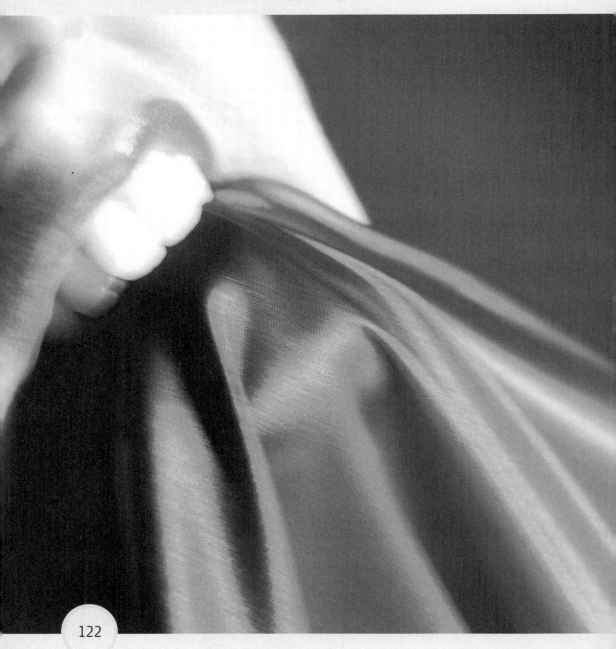

28

OH OH OH OH...oh?

It seems a little unfair that just when you no longer have to worry about becoming pregnant you may find your orgasms aren't the full-blown explosions they used to be.

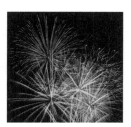

Sex during menopause has always been an issue of great debate.

Your grandmother might never have considered sex while in menopause; it was viewed with horror. Many people wondered how "elderly," infertile women dared to satisfy their sexual urges once they had lost their baby-making abilities. Menopausal women were considered sexless beings who had no business engaging in sexual activity. Menopausal women are now understood to be as feminine as they ever were, with an active sexual appetite. But, sadly, you might encounter problems with your sex life.

THE ELUSIVE ORGASM

Sometimes your orgasms are going to feel different. Instead of those long, breathy things you hear women in films having—or the ones you used to have when you were younger—these days an orgasm can be over very soon. One woman described hers as being a little solitary beat, whereas she used to have a huge throbbing sensation—so she is a bit disenchanted. You might begin to wonder if it's really

Here's an idea for you…

Dong quai, black cohosh, vitex agnus castus, and sage all help relieve the discomfort of vaginal dryness, as do dandelion leaves and oat straw. But do administer them orally. There are also estrogen and progesterone creams that are applied directly to the vagina and work quickly to lubricate the area.

worth the effort of getting worked up if your actual orgasm is nothing more than a wash-out. Another menopausal woman I know said it was better to "save them all up and have one good one instead of lots of little ones…" But what if you saved them all up and then still only had one small one?

If you have a problem having an orgasm, masturbation can help you. Extra stimulation (before you have sex with your partner) with a vibrator may be helpful. You might need rubbing or stimulation for up to an hour before having sex. Many menopausal women don't have an orgasm during intercourse. If you want an orgasm with intercourse, you or your partner may want to gently stroke your clitoris.

Defining idea…

"Clinton lied. A man might forget where he parks or where he lives, but he never forgets oral sex, no matter how bad it is."

BARBARA BUSH

There might be another problem. If you're having pain during sex—possible as your vaginal walls thin due to dropping estrogen levels—then try a natural lubricant and have sex in different positions.

NATURAL AIDS

Herbal remedies for treating various problems associated with the female reproductive
organs have been used for centuries. These
include yohimbe bark, licorice root, damiana,
saw palmetto, Siberian ginseng, histidine, vitamin B_6, and niacin. They have worked
for years in treating female hormonal needs and you might try them, as they claim
to increase libido and tone the sexual organs as well.

**IDEA 52, *How is it for you?*, is
bursting with the experiences
of women who have been
through menopause.**

*Try
another
idea...*

WITH OR WITHOUT?

Your pubic hair might begin to turn gray; there are dyes for them if you feel
strongly enough about keeping them the way they were. Or they might simply
begin to fall out—but as it's fashionable to have a Brazilian wax these days, just
think of the money you'll save. Plus, you might experience a stronger orgasm if you
get rid of your pubic hair because your clitoris can rub directly against his thrusting
pelvis and this friction is supposed to be very stimulating.

Whatever you decide, the route to finding your own menopausal orgasm will be
fun, and it shouldn't take too long before you achieve a satisfactory throb again!

*"I don't know the question but
sex is definitely the answer."*
WOODY ALLEN

*Defining
idea...*

How did it go?

Q **You can keep your sex manuals, as I have no intention whatsoever of having sex again. I don't like mixing bodily fluids and I am hugely relieved it is all over for me. I am 46, in menopause, and happily married. Am I weird not to want any sexual contact?**

A *Well, that seems pretty clear, doesn't it? If you and your husband are both happy with the situation there's no problem. But do keep in the back of your mind that a teeny bit of lovemaking can be such an intimate act at times when you might be feeling quite lonely through menopause, and it can help you feel healthy and feminine and beautiful. But no one has to make love, do they?*

Q **When I was younger, I had an affair and the sex was great between us and now each time I make love with my husband I think of my lover—and then I reach orgasm. I feel so guilty, especially since we are both in our fifties. Should I tell him?**

A *If he doesn't know about the affair then that could be why you are fantasizing about it—to keep it naughty. If he knows and you are still thinking about the other man then it might be time to figure it out. Would you like him to be thinking about another woman, especially one he had sex with, while making love to you? Unless you can share the memory and make it naughty—go very carefully—there will be trouble ahead.*

29

Want a snack?

Worried you'll feel hungry all day as soon as the word "diet" is mentioned?

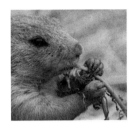

Well, it's time to get serious about your food but there is absolutely no need to starve yourself. In fact, it's just the opposite—you can graze as often as you like.

With all the information concerning diet and what you should and shouldn't be eating, you can console yourself that even though you're menopausal, a bit of what you crave really does do you good.

THE GOOD

You can munch your way through unlimited veggies—especially the leafy green types—legumes, and whole grains. Make sure you regularly eat cold-water fish such as salmon and increase your fiber intake.

Here's an idea for you...

Buy fresh foods whenever you can—if your fridge and cupboards are well stocked with good foods then you'll think twice before you grab cookies, chocolate, cake, and chips. Have good foods handy and easy to get at, and keep cookies, cake, and sweets in a tin or jar at the back so they are more difficult to get at if you think you might be tempted. Everyone will benefit if you cut out buying the junk food, and your more positive frame of mind will let them all know that the new food regime is working.

THE BAD

Cut down on alcohol, caffeine, high-fat dairy, chocolate, and anything very sugary.

THE UGLY

Downright forbidden is anything with lots of saturated fat, hydrogenated fats, non-organic animal meats, artificial sweeteners, other artificial additives, and tobacco.

Through menopause your hormone levels decline and it can be easier to put on weight. For some, this might just mean that your bust gets bigger (hooray!), but for others it will be the very last thing you want. Plus, no one wants extra fat deposits, least of all you. You also could do without those flabby upper arms and that bulging tummy. That's why it is really important to keep a check on everything you eat. Make sure the right things go in now that you are experiencing menopause and you'll reduce the chance of problems later.

When you are menopausal it's recommended that you eat small meals regularly rather than a huge meal in one sitting late at night. Try not to go without food for more than four hours at a time, so you keep blood-sugar levels stable, and drink water to keep toxins flushed out and things moving around your body.

Look at IDEA 49, *OK, but make it a small one*, for more information about drinking.

Try another idea…

Can you safely cut down on meat during menopause? Well, most nutritionists are in agreement that you can. By replacing animal proteins with plant foods such as soy products you are introducing phytoestrogens—foods that are demonstrated to have protective influences against breast and endometrial cancer. These protective foods are tofu and other soy products like miso, red beans, chickpeas, and lentils, and are great if you are experiencing menopausal hot flashes, vaginal dryness, and thinning bones. They are also known to protect against heart disease.

Hormonal imbalances can trigger sugar cravings. If that's you, then sweeten your foods with natural sugars as apple juice, citrus sweeteners, maple syrup, and Manuka honey, expensive but crammed with helpful amino acids.

Boosting your calcium intake by making sure your diet contains fewer dairy products but more foods such as leafy green vegetables, nuts, seaweed, sardines, salmon, and oysters will keep brittle bones at bay. If you can't resist dairy then make sure it's organic so you're not swamped with bovine growth hormones and antibiotics.

You are also entitled to that glass of red, white, or sparkling wine—and if it helps you relax as you enjoy preparing dinner, or if you sip

"You may have to fight a battle more than once to win it."

MARGARET THATCHER

Defining idea…

it while other people cook, then all the better. Enjoying your food, knowing that it will make you feel better, helps you have a great menopause. Food is there to balance you out. Make the most of it—experiment. Fact: You'll feel less bloated, slimmer, and sexier as soon as you ditch the junk.

How did it go?

Q   I feel as though I'm losing the fight with food. I want all of the wrong things. How can I fight the cravings?

A   *First of all, it happens to us all. It's so easy to eat the wrong foods, they are always there... At menopause a part of you would like to give in and give up, but if you can make a new diet part of your new life you will unlock a charge of vital energy. Eat colorful and beautiful foods since they contain the most antioxidants. Have total faith that what you are doing right now is the way to create feelings of safety and comfort in your body and if you lose it a couple of times, so what? Don't beat yourself up and create more stress. Ask yourself why you wanted to eat a whole package of cookies, listen to what your body tells you, then move on.*

Q   How do I cope when I am invited out to eat?

A   *There will always be something on the menu. Even if you are invited to a burger joint you could eat the veggie burger and salad. Choose items that aren't deep-fried, avoid heavy desserts and cheeses at the end of a meal, and opt for fruit instead. You'll find that if you go easy you won't suffer a hot flash, especially if you choose a light red wine and make a glass last awhile. Say no to coffee at the end of the meal and request an herb tea or hot water. Finally, enjoy yourself!*

30

Gasping for air

As you read this are you breathing through your nose or your mouth?

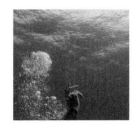

Chances are you are using your mouth and not your nose. Here's how to breathe again.

Someone told me once that we tend to breathe in a much more shallow way than we ought to, and that this could be due to our trying not to breathe in polluted air. As soon as we are in fresh air, we breathe normally—through our noses again.

The trouble is that through shallow breathing you could suffer from a lack of oxygen. This might be responsible for making you feel tired. Moreover, when you are in menopause you could be feeling extra tired as it is, so you are in for a double whammy. As soon as you feel tired, you slouch, you take in even less oxygen, and this adds to your feelings of lethargy.

Breathing through your nose is far better for you than breathing through your mouth, and those of you already taking yoga classes will be aware of the value of breathing properly. Taking time to breathe efficiently is so important through menopause.

Here's an idea for you... **Get a friend to massage your feet on a regular basis. As they begin, you can lean back and allow your breathing to find its natural rhythm. As you breathe in, imagine the oxygen reaching all of your organs and filling them with this powerful healing force. You can return the compliment—and know giving a massage to a friend in menopause will be doing her breathing good as well.**

If you live, as I do, near a main road and you know the air you are breathing isn't healthy, then buy an ionizer. These little machines are available from all large pharmacies and can be tucked away in a room unseen but they make the air clean and charge it with those negative ions. I have one in my bedroom so at least I know that when I sleep I am taking in good air to rejuvenate and heal my body and organs. Plus, oxygen is calming, and slow, deep breaths help you sleep—useful since you might find menopause has brought you bouts of insomnia. Open a window at night, whatever the temperature, and let the fresh air in.

As you lie in bed, breathe slowly to the count of ten through your nose, hold for five, and release the air to the count of ten, through your mouth. Do this five or six times each evening to induce a feeling of relaxation and to help you on your way to oxygenating your body.

Oxygen is free, it is around us day and night, and is probably one of the most important health-giving things we have at our disposal. It makes sense to get the basics right and learn to use this valuable commodity, especially through menopause when you might be feeling anxious and stressed out. A perfect antidote to that is to breathe for your health, and your menopausal health will improve no end once you get this right.

TAKE AN OXYGEN BREAK

Many of you might be stressed out because you are doing too much of the wrong thing. You are thinking too much and worrying all the time. As soon as you worry your breathing changes and becomes shallow. Then, because you are starved of oxygen, you feel ill and so you worry more. Now do you see the way the cycle works?

I think we are all in the same boat: We think too much and don't take time to play. As you relax, you breathe deeply and feel ten times better. That's why when you are on a vacation you are revitalized and recharged, but the minute you return to work the old stressors are there so your breathing tightens and oxygen intake is restricted.

How about taking time each day to catch your breath? Treat a part of every day as though it is a vacation. Recapture the feeling you had on your best-ever vacation and every day go to that place mentally for just a couple of minutes. Really be there. Breathe that place in, right to the bottom of your lungs. Breathe out and allow menopause to take a backseat for a moment. Take this moment to relax and get a breath of fresh air. Return to whatever you were doing reenergized and ready to continue on with your day.

See IDEA 15, *Don't you just love water?*, for ways of cleansing and utilizing another of nature's gifts during menopause.

Try another idea...

"Breathe. Let go and remind yourself that this very moment is the only one you know you have for sure."

OPRAH WINFREY

Defining idea...

How did it go? **Q** **I smoke but lately I feel like I want to quit. Will giving up help me during menopause?**

      A   *Absolutely. Smoking starves your body of oxygen. You probably know that your lungs are struggling for air with each cigarette, but so is your blood supply. Your coronary arteries supply oxygen to your heart and, through smoking, they, too, become clogged. You have probably seen pictures of smokers' lungs coated with a black tarry substance. Not much oxygen is going to get through that. Give up now and give your whole body the chance to breathe. It will make menopause so much easier to handle.*

31

Supplements—a waste of money?

If you're like me, you probably have a bathroom cabinet stuffed full of vitamins, minerals, and supplements you forget to take...

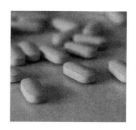

You may even have forgotten what they were for in the first place. Here's some guidance.

I discovered that some supplements need a few weeks before they kick in, so if you are only taking them for a week or two and then stop because you haven't felt any immediate benefit, you are wasting your money hand over fist. Give them a chance.

Now, if you do suspect the supplement you bought isn't working, you can check out its efficacy by doing the simple vinegar test:

- Place your supplement in a glass of warm vinegar.
- Stir it every few minutes for about half an hour.

If the supplement has not dissolved then you can safely bet it isn't being absorbed completely during digestion and is leaving your body untouched. If you do get this negative reaction, and the supplement is a waste of time, then write to the

Here's an idea for you... **Sprouted flaxseed powder can be added to cakes, soups, sprinkled over salads and vegetables, and is a delicious way to ensure you get all the omega-3 your body needs. It's also an excellent source of iron and iodine as well as containing the eight essential amino acids. It is an easily absorbed, easily taken food that you won't want to live without once you've taken it. Hunt it down online.**

manufacturer and ask for an explanation. You pay enough for supplements so they really should work.

Although nutritionists often dismiss supplements, they do have a role to play as long as they are not a substitute for a healthy diet but are, as their name suggests, a supplement to it.

Choosing a supplement can be daunting. Broadly, what you are looking for throughout menopause are these:

■ Up to 2,000 milligrams of vitamin C daily spread in small amounts over a day so you have a constant supply in your system. Vitamin C supports your blood vessels as well as your adrenal glands (for hormonal activity).

- Then, for your bones and for metabolizing calcium and your vitamin C, you should take 300–400 milligrams of magnesium every day. Again, divide the dose into smaller units and take it over the course of a day. You excrete magnesium whenever you pee, and more when you are under stress—highly likely when you are menopausal.

Read IDEA 29, *Want a snack?*, for ways to continue on the straight and narrow.

Try another idea...

- Zinc. 15–30 milligrams daily is good as well; it helps with the absorption of calcium supplements and supports your blood-sugar levels.

You need essential fatty acids to keep your hair, skin, and nails healthy. They're also beneficial for aching joints, forgetfulness, and breast pain. Your body can't make them, so you need to incorporate them in your diet. You get a good supply in some oils, nuts and seeds, tahini (sesame seed paste), and oily fish—mackerel, sardines, salmon, and tuna. Here's a basic guide.

- Monounsaturated fats are found in olive oil, rapeseed and groundnut oils, walnuts, and avocados.
- Polyunsaturated fats are also good for your well-being and health. There are omega-3 fatty acids, which lower your blood pressure, improve energy levels, help keep skin soft, and prevent heart problems. Omega-3 is found in linseed (also known as flaxseed), pumpkin seeds, oily fish, and dark green leafy vegetables; fish oil supplements are also a great source.
- The other polyunsaturated group you need is omega-6. They help keep your blood thin, reduce inflammation, and ease joint pain. They are found in sunflower and corn oils, soy, evening primrose, starflower, and borage.

"Any little bit of experimenting in self-nurturance is very frightening for most of us."

JULIE CAMERON, author

Defining idea...

You can buy supplements online, and many websites offer bargains—two for the price of one, for example—which are well worth checking out.

How did it go?

Q   I want to know more about the antioxidants the magazines go on about. What are they, and should I be taking some throughout menopause?

A   *Antioxidants are possibly the most important of all the nutrients because they neutralize free radicals. Free radicals are formed by exposure to such things as tobacco smoke, alcohol, insecticides, radiation, chemicals in the home or at work (chlorine, new carpeting, air fresheners, etc.), and even excessive amounts of sunlight. Other causes are a high-fat diet, deep-fried foods, or strenuous exercise. The effect of free-radical attacks is called oxidative damage, and as we age, our bodies become less effective at combating this—leading to signs of aging. Antioxidants slow down the aging process, as well as protect against heart disease. Make sure you eat between five to eight servings of fruits and vegetables every day. If your diet prohibits this for any reason then try taking an antioxidant supplement.*

Q   I supplement my diet with vitamin and mineral pills but they make me feel quite nauseous. Is there a "right" time to take them?

A   *Always take your supplements with a meal, as they are absorbed more efficiently when taken with food. Plus, if you take them on an empty stomach the effect can be as you describe—so always take them when you are eating, or immediately afterward.*

32

It's her hormones...

To take or not to take, that is the question.

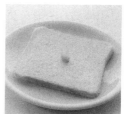

Women tend to be very neatly divided into those who swear by HRT and those who would not touch it with a ten-foot pole.

I only tried HRT for a month or so but was acutely uncomfortable with it. I was irritated by this little patch stuck on my hip, so much so that even in the bath I never felt quite naked. Then one morning my husband woke up and it was stuck to his back. I knew it was a sign telling me to try something else. I know women who have tried HRT and loved it, while others have come off it because they were concerned that the possible risks associated with HRT weren't worth the payoff from any benefits they were experiencing.

SO WHAT IS THE CURRENT HRT ADVICE?

Of course, I, like you, want a healthy body that will last me for the rest of my life as well as wanting to find ways to deal with increasing and unwanted symptoms, aches, and those funny pains that seem to appear and that I assume are linked to menopause. If you are interested in knowing more about or are considering taking

Here's an idea for you... **If you are going to try natural alternatives to HRT, before you make an appointment, make sure your practitioner is a reputable one. You can do this by asking a practitioner which professional organization they belong to and whether or not they are properly registered practitioners. Do some checking.**

HRT then the best thing to do is to take some questions to your doctor who will be able to advise you.

Good questions to ask are:

- What would I gain from taking HRT?
- Do you recommend estrogen only or a progesterone/estrogen therapy? Why?
- What form will it take? Why?
- What are the known and suspected side effects?
- How long do you think I will be taking this for? Will my symptoms return once I stop taking HRT?
- Can I review the situation with you after six months, or earlier if I have any worries or concerns about being on it?
- What alternatives do you suggest?

ALTERNATIVES TO HRT

For those of you who might like to try a natural way to deal with menopausal symptoms there are foods and supplements you can take. Always check with the practitioner or person selling you the product that it is right for you.

One supplement you could investigate is maca. Maca is a tuberous plant grown at 14,000 feet or more above sea level in the Peruvian mountains. It is an ideal substitute for HRT, as it works to stimulate the endocrine system, enabling it to deliver hormones itself in the correct quantity and proportion. It has no known side effects and claims have been made that, through being encouraged to continue its own hormone production, the body does not become lazy and reliant on external hormone delivery systems.

Go to IDEA 20, *Do you like thunder and lightning?*, for other ways to regulate menopausal symptoms.

Try another idea...

"If women are supposed to be less rational and more emotional at the beginning of our menstrual cycle when the female hormone is at its lowest level, then why isn't it logical to say that, in those few days, women behave the most like the way men behave all month long?"

GLORIA STEINEM

Defining idea...

141

Soy is one of many phytoestrogens that will benefit you through menopause. Phytoestrogens can mimic estrogen, and can help stabilize your fluctuating hormones throughout menopause. As always, though, check that your source is organic, because organic means it won't have been genetically modified. There's a lot of GM soy in the marketplace.

Other foods rich in phytoestrogens are:

- Kidney beans, mung beans, chickpeas, peas, and lentils
- Linseed, sunflower seeds, pumpkin seeds, and sesame seeds
- Rice, oats, barley, and wheat
- Broccoli, rhubarb, potatoes, celery, radishes, fennel, apples, and carrots
- Green tea
- Sprouting beans like alfalfa
- Soy products like soybean curd (tofu), soy milk, miso, and tempeh

Q **I'm worried because I live such a busy life and don't have the time for a more natural approach to menopause. For instance, I know I won't remember to eat all those phytoestrogen foods or take lots of pills throughout the day. Is there something easy I can choose without resorting to HRT?**

How did it go?

A *If you opt for HRT you don't have to think about menopause at all. Now, it's certainly true that a holistic approach means being vigilant every day for the rest of your life about your diet and making sure you are taking the right foods to suit you. But this longer route will have an impact on every aspect of your life and the benefits will be forever. There are supplements you can take to accommodate your busy lifestyle and one particularly good one is Natural HRT, which claims to relieve hot flashes, night sweats, sleep disturbances, mood swings, headaches, loss of libido, vaginal dryness, and anxiety. It contains soy, red clover, vitex angus castus, dong quai, black cohosh, natural vitamin E, and vitamin B_{12}.*

Q **I have been thinking about visiting a Chinese herbalist about my menopause. Might this be a good idea?**

A *Chinese herbal medicine is one of the oldest forms of medicine and has developed a particular formula for menopause based on thousands of years of experience. The ingredients chosen work to adjust the yin–yang balance and regulate hormone levels. There have been claims it could be the best herbal formula in the world and has none of the side effects of HRT.*

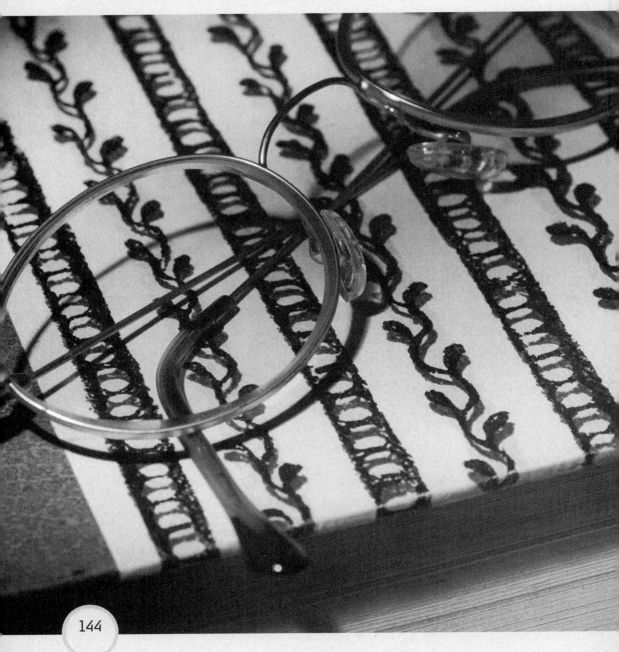

33

Make a note of it

Have you ever considered keeping a journal of your experiences as you go through menopause?

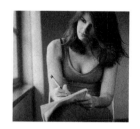

Keeping a journal or diary is a creative way to express your thoughts, your feelings, and your emotions. And, importantly, it's yours!

That means it's private, it's yours to own and to keep. Let's face it, so many times in your life, your time and your energy is called upon by others. As a woman, you care for the needs of other people, often putting those needs above your own. But menopause is a personal journey, so why not record it? Keeping a journal during menopause is not only a record of your changes, your achievements, and your relationships, you can also use it to see how you've felt, what you've learned, and what menopause means to you. It's a tool to help you. A journal could be just for you, or you might like to let your husband or partner or best friend read it. Or maybe your daughter, knowing that one day, she, too, will be menopausal. You will be passing on your newfound knowledge and wisdom to her and she will benefit from what you have to say.

Here's an idea for you...

You may find that you have vivid and colorful dreams during menopause. Write them down. Not to analyze or worry about, but for you to enjoy the marvel and wonder of your imagination, even when you are asleep.

Because the journal is yours, it's up to you when you write in it, how you write, and what you say. It's a highly personalized account of one of the greatest changes to celebrate in your life. Did you know that Michelangelo, Virginia Woolf, and Van Gogh all kept journals? As you go through menopause, writing will not only fulfill those creative desires you have, but you'll also realize you are teaching yourself about yourself. You'll be able to see how you make decisions, how you react to things, and come to understand what is important about menopause.

So begin by choosing a special book that you will want to write in. Choose a notebook that you like the look of. It could have a colorful cover, or one that's easily cleaned. It could be a leather-bound or spiral-bound book. It might have lined or plain paper in it, or even colored paper. It can be a notebook with illustrations that you love—flowers, forests, or animals. Buy yourself a special pen or colored pens if you like, it's up to you. You could put in special photos or tickets or leaflets that mean something to you, even a pressed flower... Don't limit your journal to just writing. You could sketch or draw in it. Remember that it's yours and nobody can find fault with anything you want to put or do in it. The possibilities are endless.

Here are a few tips on how to make keeping a journal easier for yourself:

- Try to focus on your feelings and thoughts about things. The journal is not just about what you did and when.
- Make yourself comfortable when you begin to write. This can be in your favorite chair or in the garden on a warm day or evening.
- Collect your thoughts, be calm, and take a deep breath before you begin. But don't think too hard about what you write, just let it happen.
- Start with little notes if you think you may have a lot to say—that way you won't forget and find yourself rushing back to it later.
- Write freely, write down whatever comes to mind. The more you do, the easier it will be.
- Try to set aside a special time for your writing, a time when you won't be disturbed or have to rush off to shop or cook.
- Get yourself in the right mood. Maybe you might want to put on some gentle music or have soft lighting on around you. Maybe you will find yourself needing silence—in that case, make sure you're alone.

Keep track of your feelings. See IDEA 51, *Am I going crazy?*, for more help and reassurance.

Try another idea...

You may be surprised to find out how many people find that keeping a journal can relieve the stresses and tensions of being menopausal. You know how quickly time flies by, how you forget many things because life is so busy and hectic. Writing is therapeutic as well. It will help you to put things in perspective and will relieve tension as you record this important period in your life. It will help you come to terms with what is happening to you. It will be a pleasurable experience. So keeping a journal is simple and easy, it is fun, and you will no doubt find yours satisfying to write in, and to read over.

"I never travel without my diary. One should always have something sensational to read on the train."

OSCAR WILDE

Defining idea...

147

How did it go?

Q **The journal idea sounds interesting but I don't really have the time to write every day. What should I do?**

A   *Although you may want to put a date on each entry, you do not have to write in it on a daily basis. Sometimes you will find yourself writing more on one day than on others and that's OK; the frequency is up to you. But remember, the more you write, the more you will want to write, so it doesn't matter if you find it difficult at first.*

Q **I still can't spell very well and I don't really know where to use all of those grammatical things! Can I really do this?**

A   *Of course you can! Remember, you don't have to be a professional to write. Spelling, grammar, language—none of that matters here. Your journal is a powerful and creative thing, a space for you to reflect on how you feel. It is about your innermost thoughts and emotions, a focus for self-expression and self-exploration.*

34

Keep it in the family

To tell or not to tell? Let them know what you are going through. Or, keep quiet and keep them guessing.

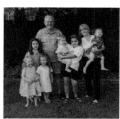

What you tell them and how much is up to you, but it might be a good idea to let them know that things are a little different these days now that you are menopausal.

Is it time to tell them that you are menopausal? Do you want them to know? It's not that as soon as you hit the change you stop being a mom, lover, best friend—far from it. It just means that your mothering skills kick up a notch and in a way become even more meaningful. As a lover you are more empathetic and understand your partner's need to spend time alone reflecting.

You, through menopause, are offering your family—and to some extent your friends—the chance to change as well. They are witnessing something going on that is both ordinary and extraordinary, and your menopause will affect them. Explain your feelings and needs to them. Maybe you could ask them what they feel they need at this time as well, and whether they feel alienated from you. Would

Here's an idea for you...

This sounds crazy but why don't you hold a little "coming of age" party for family and close friends so you can all celebrate your new life? It needn't be an elaborate affair but make it special, something to mark the occasion in a way you can laugh about it, talk about it, have a drink about it. A party would let everyone know your life isn't anything like over and that you have renewed energy and want to share your new life with others. Choose your favorite music and food, dance, and be as excited as you possibly can. By being open and sharing, you are letting others into your life in a big way.

they like to be able to support you more? In what way can they help you get through? How can you all help each other get the best out of menopause?

Everyone is a bit wary of change so they won't be relishing the idea of a new you, or even a slightly "changed" you for that matter, and so they might not like the fact you are menopausal. They know it means something different but won't be sure how different. Maybe you could spend a little time telling them how menopause has affected you and they might not feel so threatened. They might appreciate that you have shared it with them.

It could be that you want some space and more privacy, after having had your personal space invaded for years. One woman told me she even felt guilty about having a lock put on her bathroom door so she could bathe or shower without being interrupted and that her husband took it very personally. He didn't understand that it wasn't so much about not wanting him barging in whenever he wanted to ask her something, but that she needed that time to herself. Most of you have shared bathroom time with kids in the past, and if you still don't have a lock on that door…well, now is the time. You only need a few minutes of undisturbed privacy every day to feel a whole lot better and by now, with menopause, you have earned it. Anyway, everything can wait until you have soaked, taken off your face mask, and done your legs. It really is not so much to ask and will make you feel a whole lot better.

IDEA 33, *Make a note of it*, will encourage you to acknowledge your feelings during menopause.

Try another idea…

Privacy might be something you notice coming high on your agenda more and more as you travel through stages of menopause. You do need time to simply "be" and maybe if your family doesn't realize what you are going through they won't understand your need for it.

It can be difficult spluttering those first few words about being at the start of menopause. Some of you might be with partners who won't even realize you have been menopausal for quite a while. Menopause is not their fault, and unless you tell it how it is, how are they expected to know what to do? It's new for you and it's new for them, too. You will all be different when it's over.

"Everything in life that we really accept undergoes a change."

KATHERINE MANSFIELD

Defining idea…

151

How did it go?

Q **My best friend is menopausal—in fact, we started at about the same time. But she and I totally differ in our approach to it and are almost falling out over what to take and what not to take, like HRT. What's the best solution?**

A *Sometimes we get competitive about the way we deal with aspects of life. There are many options, so explain to your friend that there isn't just one "best way" and try not to react if she says she knows best. Focus on how she is coping and, if you can, swallow your pride and thank her for the information she gives you. You never know—in the end she could even ask you for your advice.*

Q **I feel very embarrassed at having to admit to my younger partner that I had my last period over a year ago. He thinks I still have regular periods and now I do not know whether to admit the truth. I am scared he'll think I'm growing old. I'm 52. Should I tell him?**

A *Menopause can strike at 35 or 60 so he must know it's a possibility, at least, that at 52 you could be menopausal. Take a deep breath and tell him. Explain your doubts and fears and then you can get on with your life. He'll probably wonder what on earth all the fuss was about.*

35

Focus on the good stuff

If anything is guaranteed to make you feel worse it's continually harping about how bad you're feeling or how miserable the world is now that you're menopausal.

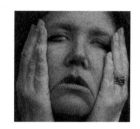

Of course, some days you might be feeling like death warmed over—but haven't you always had days like that anyway?

On those bad days, or even on good days, why not indulge yourself and take to your bed for the day if you're able to do so? Take a book or a few magazines, the radio, something to eat, and jump back into bed. Once in a while it is the greatest thing to do and, apart from being able to snooze, you will get those "thinking" moments when your mind goes backward and forward through time recalling moments, incidents, people, places, and things that have happened in your life. Sometimes this alone can be enough to bring you back to a positive frame of mind and make you feel good about the world again.

If you are really down then there might be something you need to address seriously. One way to deal with anything making you feel blocked through menopause might be to see a really good reflexologist or herbalist who will be equipped to help you deal with issues that are preventing you from moving forward in your life.

Here's an idea for you... **Try a retreat somewhere in the countryside. Just you and a few days being taken care of without any of the trappings of the outside world could be all you need to make you feel fabulous again.**

Don't book the first one you find. Ask on the phone about how they work and how many sessions you are likely to need, as well as how much it will cost. Sometimes just a couple of sessions will be all that's required to get back on track again. If you have to make difficult decisions at this time, and your menopause will make you challenge every aspect of your life, then it is always good to talk to someone else about what your choices are and ask them to help you understand why you need to make these changes.

Depression can be a sign that the body wants you to move to a different place mentally. Instead of dwelling on "you," it can really help to get out there and dwell on others. Sometimes the depression will lift of its own accord, making you feel valued and positive again.

Apart from a massage—guaranteed to make you feel better for a short time at least—you could scrutinize your diet. Check that you are eating wholesome foods and that you are eating regularly. You are exercising and getting fresh air at least a couple of times a week and you don't sit at home in front of the box every night, do you? Nothing will make you feel worse than watching someone else's life every night rather than getting on with your own now that you are in menopause. Your body demands you give it attention and watching television every night is no way to relax day in, day out. Watch a film, a good documentary, and rubbish now and then—but if it becomes a habit it drains you of your life.

You could also try meditation to give you a clearer vision of where you want to be. Meditation allows you to discover the silence, the stillness, which creates an inner peacefulness and renews your energy for everyday life. As recognized benefits of meditation increase to include focus, creativity, vital energy, enhanced learning, and performance, deeper self-awareness and a happier, healthier lifestyle, it is becoming a popular practice.

Take a look at IDEA 34, *Keep it in the family.* Letting them know what you are going through should help them understand your needs at this time.

Try another idea…

Menopause wants you to reclaim your life and if you slump you will hit a negative state, for sure. No one wants to moan all the time, least of all you, and if you feel really grim on an off day then make a joke about it. Laughter is a great cure—we all love someone who is willing and able to laugh at themselves, especially through menopause.

If you can find it in you to stay positive when you are negative then you have found the key to happiness, and the way to get you through almost any situation. Knowing you can rely on yourself to get you through a negative day is half the solution. Preventing that negative day is the other half.

"It's a funny thing about life; if you refuse to accept anything but the best, you very often get it."
SOMERSET MAUGHAM

Defining idea…

How did it go?

Q **I have tried to stay positive through menopause but sometimes I find it really hard not to sink into gloom. Where am I going wrong?**

A *If you think you are suffering from depression then seek help from your doctor who may refer you for counseling. You could also get more rest, give yourself "me time," and keep a note of what triggers your depression: The solution could well be found therein.*

Q **My friend moans about everything and she makes me feel worse. What should I do?**

A *She could be unaware she is having such a lowering effect on you. Either ignore her moans and change the subject or try to get her to lighten up a little. Failing that, you could go to the movies together, where she won't have much chance to talk to you, or simply let her moan away but tell yourself it is not going to have any impact on you at all. Use her moans as a way of measuring your own personal growth. As soon as the moaning has stopped touching you, hey presto, you are in control.*

36

Musical madness

Do you feel you are struggling to "find your voice"?

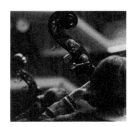

It's common around menopause to think that you aren't being listened to, and your world can turn into a strange and silent place where you aren't being heard.

Each of us has a voice that is as unique as our DNA. Your voice will not resonate, sound like, or emit the same vibration as any other person's on the planet. It is always important that each of us "finds our own voice" but especially so during menopause. Your voice is the expression of your life experience, your thoughts, emotions, and feelings. But the tension and stresses of being menopausal can create blockages in the way you express yourself and you might find your voice becomes thinner and less powerful. You might not even want to be heard after a while.

Through developing your full vocal expression, you are empowering yourself and will regain health, confidence, and joy in your life again. One way of doing this is by singing. Through learning to create a flexible vocal singing range, you learn to breathe properly and as soon as you do, oxygen flows freely throughout your body again and your general well-being is enhanced.

There are so many therapies out there to help you "find your voice" and these work through a variety of means, so do a quick search online. The one I attended, given by Jill Purce, was a weekend course and I was terrified I might have to sing in front of everyone.

A teacher once said that I had a flat singing voice and that put me off ever singing in public again, so I was nervous as I sat waiting for the class to begin. Jill started by getting us to sit with our mouths hanging open, which can't have looked very pretty. We relaxed our jaws and shoulders simply through sitting comfortably. Honestly, within minutes I felt tension leaving my body in waves. Then we had to adjust our breathing to allow breath to lightly brush against our vocal cords. It sounded so eerie but as I progressed and made that sound stronger I produced amazing, comforting sounds.

We were shown how to deepen our breathing further and let the sounds fly. Once that happened, I just rode the waves of harmonics, and soon it seemed that the overtones were emanating from my whole body. It helped that Jill was of menopausal age, and the feeling I had very strongly was that this is something we menopausal women should all practice on an almost daily basis. If you see a chanting or singing course advertised I urge you to try it out. It will change your life, without a doubt.

Here's an idea for you... **Join a choir and learn to free your voice again. Explain that you are shy or can't sing and they will tell you everyone can sing. I don't agree with that, but I like the idea that we all have a voice and can train it to make it sound a whole lot better.**

Tape yourself and listen to your own voice. I was really shocked at how I disliked my voice when I first heard it; I reacted in the same way as whenever I see bad photographs of myself. But if you listen to your own voice it helps you identify what other people hear when you speak, and offers you the chance to change it.

See IDEA 22, *Powerful tools, words*, to discover more about menopause and how to influence your life through the language you speak.

Try another idea...

Here are some small changes you can make to strengthen your voice:

- Chant quietly to yourself each evening with your eyes closed so you can become familiar with your voice.
- When you feel comfortable, experiment a little with your vocal range and feel the notes resonate throughout your body.

You will honestly feel a million times better. Look after your voice throughout menopause and it will stay a friend for the rest of your life.

You could use music differently, of course. You might decide that a blast on the piano might work for you, or learning to play the guitar. Some menopausal women I know in Scotland have formed a rock band and play at charity bashes—all of them are in their forties and fifties. They use the garage for rehearsals and are from non-musical back-grounds. It's created a stir but they're having lots of fun and each member of the band says she has increased her level of self-confidence.

"All my concerts had no sounds in them: they were completely silent. People had to make up their own music in their minds!"

YOKO ONO

Defining idea...

How did it go? **Q** **My daughter listens to very different music from the kind I like. Hers is ugly and she plays it at top volume. I am forever bellowing, "Turn that thing down." I used to be able to cope but now that I'm menopausal it really grates on my nerves. Can you help?**

A *Couldn't you suggest (or even buy her) a set of headphones? She could play her music loudly and won't offend anyone. I think you need to tell her about your menopause and that you are more sensitive now. And, of course, there are the neighbors. Most people say that their biggest fear is living next to noisy neighbors. Tell your daughter quite firmly that she has to wear the headset or turn it down.*

Q **I am in an amateur operatic society and only stay because I am in love with the conductor, but he is gay. I feel like a teenager but no one else comes close to him for humor, sensitivity, and beauty. What can I do?**

A *It sounds good from here. You must spend quite a lot of time together as it is. Cultivate the friendship and carry on enjoying the singing. You might not get your man as a lover, but you'll have a great time improving your singing voice and flirting with him. A little flirting while you are menopausal is no bad thing, anyway.*

37

Unresolved matters

The past has a powerful way of controlling the present.

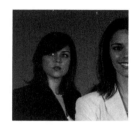

Dealing with the past when you are menopausal is important—even if you're just letting go of it.

You might find yourself thinking about the past more and more once you are menopausal, and especially about all those people you had but have now lost in your life. Major losses, for instance, can rule our lives for years with feelings of helplessness, confusion, and overwhelming sadness. If your losses are not resolved through menopause, they can drain you of energy and interfere with your ability to live fully in the present.

LOSSES

Spend some quiet time thinking of someone close you loved but have lost, some-one you might not have mourned over properly when they died. Be prepared for it to hurt and then write them a letter as though they were still alive, telling them you love them and thanking them for all of their love and nurturing, or explaining why you hurt them as you did. Keep the letter somewhere safe and add to it when you feel the desire to speak with them. If you make a special time for this then you are dealing with the past in a powerful way, but it is not holding you back in your life.

Here's an idea for you... **Call on the help of a loved one if there is a secret you have held in your closet for a very long time and you feel frightened about bringing it out in the open and telling those you love and who love you. When you know the time has come to face it, then ask their advice about how to proceed. It is very scary but very important, and if you feel you have to deal with it then you must do so. Afterward there could be some fallout but you will experience a sense of freedom and those around you will value your honesty—no matter how difficult they might find whatever you have said.**

Then make the decision to move on. Make the supreme effort to let them go so that you're not going to spend your life under the spell of old issues and past relationships, living so much in the past that you fail to connect with the experiences of the present.

UNRESOLVED ISSUES

Face up to these. It can be really scary to have to deal with something you'd rather not, but once you break through this barrier of fear, you will have a new energy and be able to live your life again as a whole woman. It will feel as though you have stepped out of a prison cell. Seek out people who can be trusted and who can listen well. During times of dealing with unresolved matters, you need to talk to someone to share the intense thoughts and feelings you experience when you are alone.

Your unresolved matter might involve another person and you could well find that menopause makes you dream of this person or think about them so much that you have nowhere else to go but to seek them out and work it out. Do it, even if the event happened twenty years ago. If you need to apologize for something you have done in the past, then now is exactly the right time.

If you have been escaping the past by ignoring your relationship, then IDEA 39, *Do you still love him?*, might help you face it again.

Try another idea…

We all travel better when we travel light and dealing with unresolved issues means dumping clogged-up emotions—and can be the road to your personal freedom through menopause. What is important is that you deal with the matter in your own way: Either write it down, express it verbally, or ask for advice about what to do. Your menopausal wisdom will help you decide. Then make the decision to move on. You cannot change the past, but you can change your attitude toward it.

EMPTY NESTS

Finally, if you have kids, the empty nest syndrome often hits at about the same time as your menopause, so having watched your children grow into adulthood, you might feel that you have lost part of your old sense of identity and purpose. To cling to the past and your old parental role is to invite depression as well as conflict. This fear of no longer being an active mom is an unresolved issue and one many menopausal women experience. Again, talking it through can help.

"If you do not tell the truth about yourself, you cannot tell it about other people."
VIRGINIA WOOLF

Defining idea…

How did it go?

Q   **I was caught shoplifting when I was 16, and again at the age of 20. I was so angry when one of my children was caught doing the same five years ago but now I feel so guilty I never shared my experience with her, and fear she will never forgive me for not doing so when she needed me. It's really bothering me. Is it too late to tell her?**

A   *Mistakes are a part of everyone's life and we all learn not only from making them but also from trying not to repeat them. If your daughter brings up her experience again then there is an excellent opportunity for you to let her know how terrifying it is to be caught—and how scary it is to have to admit to others what you have done. That way she will know that she can tell her kids sooner rather than later, and you will have explained to her why you never said anything before.*

Q   **I know my partner is hiding something but he won't tell me what it is other than to say it is in the past. Since my menopause started I have wanted a closer relationship with him and feel this is driving us apart. Can I do anything?**

A   *It can be difficult waiting for a loved one to reveal something but you cannot force him. Explain you want to know what it is and then leave him alone to tell you in his own time. Tend to your own life.*

38

Looking back to the future

We all slip into the wonderful world of recollection when we are with family or old friends. There's nothing nicer than a shared past to talk about.

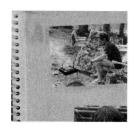

The past seems to be only yesterday though, doesn't it? I find that a bit scary~ I think my gran used to say something like that to me...

Menopause is a lovely place to be when you want to think about people you knew, places you visited, and things you did. When you are having one of those lonely menopausal moments the best company there is can be in the past. It is stimulating, lively, and emotional and will help you pass a few moments in an emotional haze. I love getting the old photo album out for this—it makes me cry each time I see pictures of my deceased mom and dad, my siblings as cute little toddlers, and, like you, I wonder where the time went. I can't believe I am almost as old as the old aunt we used to go and visit. I thought she was ancient.

It's a funny thing about aging and menopause, isn't it? I don't think we look anything like our mothers used to at this age. But, as with most things

Here's an idea for you...

If someone from the past still has the power to make you feel angry even though you no longer have contact with that person then you are stuck in a negative time-travel module. That person still holds power over you and is stealing precious energy from you. The irony is that they have no idea they are still causing you grief. Take time out to consciously let go of this person and the grip they have over you. You need to forgive them, confront them, or write a letter to yourself letting this person go once and for all. Then burn the letter and all the associations you have with this person.

emotional, you have to pack the albums away again and come back to the present. It's nice to see the world of the past through rose-colored glasses but the idea now is to get you used to the skin you are in right now and to make this the best time for your life. How?

Well, you can take the very best things from the past and incorporate them into your life if you really liked them enough. For instance, I had an aunt who had the most glorious dressing table and it seemed to have crystal vases of roses on it all year round. It was oak and on it sat a silver hairbrush and comb and one of those handheld mirrors. I thought I was a film star every time I looked into that mirror and I would pout and kiss and do things with my hair. It kept me entertained for hours whenever I stayed there.

When I married I never really considered a dressing table like that, but when I started menopause I wanted one. I found one in an antique market and bought it. I smothered it in little silver trays, pearls, perfume bottles, old photograph frames; a friend bought me a dressing table set and I pick roses whenever I can. It is my idea of heaven. Why this should have hit me when menopause began, I have no idea, but now this dressing table is a comfort and a place I love to adorn and keep beautiful. I no longer pout in the mirror, though sometimes I recall the little girl who did. I adore this little piece of furniture and that corner of the bedroom is very much mine.

Check where you hang on to outmoded feelings about money. Read IDEA 43, *Money makes the world go round...*

Try another idea...

Maybe you could find a way to connect with a part of your past that you found really beautiful and comforting. You might have seen a painting, or a glass you recall someone drinking from, that will connect you in a loving way to the past. A woman I know has a collection of Victorian nightgowns because she says her old aunt used to wear one. Another now only drinks tea from a china cup, and it's made from leaves in a proper teapot. Both these women acquired these habits when they were menopausal. When you are, it all feels extra poignant. What better way to acknowledge the power and beauty of the past than to bring part of it into the future?

"The past is not a package one can lay away."

Defining idea...

EMILY DICKINSON

How did
it go?

Q **I'm horrified to think about some of the things I said and did in the past. I keep going back to the awful things I did. I was a jerk and don't know how to get over the fact. What can I do?**

A *The past has gone and so might have half the people you dread remembering you. Let go of the past—as simple as that. Each time it wants to invade your life, ask it firmly to leave. You don't need anyone's approval for the person you were or weren't. Also remember a lot of the past is subjective—the people you mention might have no idea what you are talking about. Let it go.*

Q **My partner gets very jealous when I mention the past and we end up fighting about it. He knows I am menopausal and a little sentimental at the moment but how can I stop these fights?**

A *Try not to let him bully you about the past. Explain the past has happened and you are who you are because of it. Ask him about his past and let him see you aren't scared to listen to him talk about it. Tell him the past is no threat, as it is gone.*

39

Do you still love him?

Everyone wants to stay in love, but why do some relationships make it, while others don't? Why does the love in some relationships flourish, when it gets buried in others?

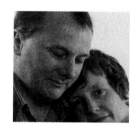

Is there a right time to leave your partner and do you have to wait until you are in screaming fights with each other?

Let's begin with a few questions.

- Is your relationship a nourishing and nurturing one?
- Do you look forward to his opinions about the things you ask him?
- Do you still chat, laugh, and cry together?
- Have you helped move each other forward through your life together?
- Do you still say you love him?
- Do you kiss?
- Are you satisfying each other's physical and spiritual needs?

Many relationships end because one or both partners can no longer communicate with the other. So, in asking whether you still love him, you are being asked to

Here's an idea for you… **Take a vacation on your own and discover how you get along without any of the familiar people around you. It needn't be anywhere exotic; a few days will be enough to allow a new rhythm in to your life and being away will encourage you to have a deeper understanding about your relationship with your partner.**

look at yourself as well as your relationship. "Do I still love him?" means knowing what love is now that you are menopausal and whether your definitions of love and relationships have changed. If you are living in a dead-end relationship you will only feel worse about yourself if you stay, and you will have to face up to the options available to you both at some point.

A friend of mine, in the full swing of menopause, left her partner of fifteen years and she says it was the most difficult thing she ever undertook in her life. She described their last moment together and I wanted to weep. She pecked him on his cheek and said she caught his familiar smell, and noticed his wedding ring was still on his finger. She felt him press against her and she could have told him it was all a ghastly mistake and tried to make it work again. That night she wanted him back and she howled. She missed him like crazy for weeks and said she felt numb and truly doubted she had done the right thing in insisting they split up. Everything was difficult. She found it hard sleeping during menopause as it was, but sleeping in an apartment without her man in bed with her was impossible. She wanted to call him each time she needed a shelf put up or a job done to the car. She says it was all the little things she found most traumatic. She seriously thought she had made a huge mistake.

It wasn't until some months later, when she realized she was starting to sort her life out, that she knew she had done the right thing. Her menopausal symptoms actually eased up a little and she began to see the forest for the trees. She began enjoying cooking for herself and eating when she wanted to eat. She found she was more open to ideas and to meeting new people and eventually she became the woman she always wanted to be. She doesn't blame her ex for anything, but says they had simply outgrown what had been a healthy relationship and that their life together had become resentful, full of sarcasm and put-me-downs.

Sometimes a trial separation when you are in menopause can be all it takes to get you back to falling in love with each other all over again. And the fact that you have split for a while can be a wonderful, liberating thing. Taking time to live alone lets you realize all the areas in which you have become dependent on each other and where you need to learn new skills—and the same will apply to him.

If you know, deep down, that the relationship still has that vital spark, then work to make it a success together. Your menopause will only want the best relationship so don't even try if you know it really is over.

IDEA 14, *If I love you, will you love me back?*, lets you know more about relationships and what is valuable about them. It could be useful if you have issues with your partner.

Try another idea…

"I will reveal to you a love potion, without medicine, without herbs, without any witches' magic; if you want to be loved, then LOVE."
HECATON OF RHODES, philosopher

Defining idea…

How did it go?

Q **Whenever I go to kiss my husband or hug him, he sees it as an opportunity to grab my breasts or press himself against me to let me feel he is becoming aroused. He says I should be grateful he's still interested in me. Sometimes all I want is a playful, flirty cuddle with no reference to sex whatsoever. How can I let him know?**

A *Part of me wants you to tell him to go jump off a cliff but the other part says that he is probably responding to the very mixed message all around us that women want sex, sex, sex. Perhaps he sees it as a compliment to tell you that he's "still interested," and doesn't realize it is more of an insult, actually. You'll have to tell him you are troubled by his constant references to sex, and let him know sometimes you just want to cuddle.*

Q **I still find my partner desirable but we no longer live together. I think I would like to give living together another try, as we seem to have resolved our differences. What do you suggest?**

A *If you love him and he loves you, and he knows you will need some space and time at the moment, then go for it. Make it clear, though, that whatever the reason for your split, it has to be fully resolved so that you can start fresh.*

40

Sex is a great idea

You might not always be in the mood but what counts is *when* you are in the mood.

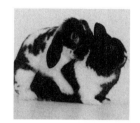

You're probably not at it 24/7 any longer; in fact, it might be more like 1/52, but it isn't quantity that counts—it's quality.

We all know that after the first lusty months of being in love, the frequency of love-making diminishes and will have halved after a couple of years. When you've been with someone for a longer period of time it is so easy to become lazy about sex and almost forget to make love. Many women head straight into menopause believing that their sex life will suffer, and they act accordingly.

During menopause, you will need touch, love, and intimacy more than before. This touch doesn't have to be full-blown intercourse; in fact, many women might prefer petting and non-penetrative sex. Once you take the time to think about what it is you would like sexually, then you know how to start communicating about sex once again.

You might find a sexy film arousing or want to experiment with sex toys and sexy underwear. Now the chances are that any kids have flown the nest, you don't have to limit your sexual activities to bedtime but can experiment with a pre-supper

Here's an idea for you…

Try sexy dates with your partner outdoors. Get into the car, go off and search for that perfect spot where you know you won't be seen and can behave like a couple of teenagers. Take a blanket if you are on the beach somewhere, or have found a field. The last thing you want is to come home covered in insect bites or scratches from stones and debris.

quickie or a lunchtime break. You can linger in bed again on a Saturday and make love until lunchtime. When you are menopausal, it is very important not to neglect your sexual needs, as they will be instrumental in helping you maintain your sense of being a woman— something you might start to feel you no longer are once menopause kicks in.

If you have lost the desire to have sex, then sometimes you might have to fake it awhile to bring it back again. When you're feeling sad, depressed, lonely, it can be hard to think that sex might be the answer, but it could be and the best way forward is to take a deep breath and just go for it. It could revitalize a flagging relationship and put you back in touch with yourself and your relationship.

Whatever your circumstances are—and I am calling all menopausal women here— your sexual appetite won't diminish just because you are menopausal. It might be more in your mind than in your body and you might need to look at or identify why you no longer want sex. Nothing will be as potent as discovering for yourself why you are struggling with a lack of libido, and although men can take Viagra for a low sex drive, I think for us menopausal women it is a different story. Of course your hormones matter, and for some women they can make a difference, but your sexuality is a many-splendored thing, and when something goes wrong you can't say "it's only hormones," or "it's only self-image," or "it's only the relationship." For menopausal women it is always a combination of factors, and a simple, Viagra-like solution will never be the answer for us.

Read IDEA 42, *Beautiful breasts*, and find out how to keep them in tip-top condition.

Try another idea…

But although saying good-bye to hormones and sex may happen in the same breath, the latest research indicates that sexual desire has less to do with menopause than it does with lifestyle and other health factors. This study found that there appeared to be no age differences with respect to frequency of sexual intercourse, or the desire for sexual activity not involving intercourse, among differing age groups. But the study concluded that the single most influential factor with regard to sexual satisfaction via intercourse was the quality of your partnership, in particular the quality of mutual respect, which becomes more important as you age. It seems most of us will want emotional closeness with our partners to bring about satisfactory physical experiences. So, if you want a good sex life, start talking and sharing each other's lives again. Your partner might be as scared as you about making the first move—but one of you has to do it. When you do, there will be no looking back.

"Don't cook. Don't clean. No man is ever going to make love to a woman because she waxed the linoleum. 'My God, the floor's immaculate. Lie down, you hot bitch.'"

JOAN RIVERS

Defining idea…

175

How did
it go?

Q **I certainly don't want another baby but nor do I want to use
contraception if it's unnecessary. So can I get pregnant now that
I am menopausal?**

A *Well, experts agree it is best to wait for two years without having a period
before you consider yourself safe if menopause started before 50. If you
were over that age when menopause started then a year is considered
safe.*

Q **Since menopause started, my sexual appetite has not dimin-
ished but my lubrication system has. I love intercourse but it
really hurts me. What can I do?**

A *There are many lubricants on the market for just this situation. Check your
local pharmacy, talk to your gynecologist, or stop by the nearest adult
store, if you're feeling brave.*

41

Lend a hand

It's not the end of the world, getting other people who live in the same house as you to chip in and help out.

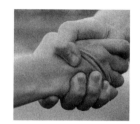

So many menopausal woman run themselves ragged trying to do everything and do all this self-discovery stuff as well.

Sometimes it can be so hard to let go of routine and habitual behavior, but during menopause you might be desperate for change. To start the process toward surviving in a family when you are in menopause, you will need to be proactive in making changes in your everyday life. These need not always cause problems. With the right attitude they can be turned into opportunities for growth for everyone.

Many menopausal women feel that their partners and/or children don't help out enough around the house. Your teenage kids like to bring all their friends over, eating the food you've just bought, and your partner might still want to watch television or have a drink after dinner. You could find yourself in exactly the same place you were before menopause started.

Here's an idea for you... It's so easy to get stuck in a rut at Christmas, doing it the same every year because that's how they all like it to be and that's how it's always been done. Fair enough, but as the family gets older they need to be given set and definite jobs to make Christmas work for everyone—including you. Make a list and make everyone commit to doing something "big" to contribute toward Christmas and let you off the hook so that you can enjoy it as well.

In addition to a general dislike of household chores, there may be significant factors influencing your family's decision not to pitch in. If you feel like a lone warrior in a war against dirt and mess in your home, it may be time to look at the reasons your family is failing to rally around. You need help now that you are in menopause and maybe you could identify why the help isn't there.

I DO IT BETTER THAN ANYONE ELSE!

If you are the type of woman who is never satisfied with other people's results, you may be teaching your house-cleaning recruits to fail. Make sure your demands are reasonable. Your family may not want to use the same method to scrub a bathtub as you do. If the bathtub gets clean and you did not have to do it, does it really matter? If your family is failing to accomplish the job, they may not fully understand what you expect—especially if you keep taking over, thinking you do it better. You are denying others the chance to help you, at a time when you need it most of all: menopause.

THEY DON'T KNOW HOW

Sometimes you may forget that jobs that are easy for you may be a mystery to the rest of your family. If they get it wrong at first, so what? It's not the end of the world.

It can be difficult to let others take over, but once you've done it a few times you'll all get the hang if it and you won't want to return to the old ways. Ever.

IDEA 2, *Warming up for the real thing*, will help you know when to start preparing people for the fact that things have to change.

Try another idea…

IT'LL GET DONE EVENTUALLY

Consider your family member's motivation for helping you. Do they have one? If you have consistently cleaned up their mess for them, then suddenly asking them to take responsibility may come as a shock. Soften the blow by holding a family meeting and let them come up with ideas for helping.

MY PARTNER IS TOO BUSY TO HELP ME

If your partner is too busy to help, then you need to limit what you do until you can get together to discuss the best way to free you up a little. Explain to your partner that this is serious and the time has come to change your life. Ask them what they think they might do in order to make your own life, and the lives of those around you, better.

"It is only when we truly know and understand that we have a limited time on earth—and that we have no time of knowing when ours is up—that we will begin to live each day to the fullest, as if it was the only one we had."

ELIZABETH KÜBLER-ROSS, author and pioneer of the hospice movement

Defining idea…

How did it go?

Q **I am a control freak and I know it. I have two kids in their twenties and they both live at home, but I'm resentful because I want space to myself now. Our house is very small and I still end up doing the housework and shopping, on the whole. I love them both dearly and don't want to hurt them. What should I do?**

A *If they're students it's likely they'll move once their studies are over but otherwise you might have to make broad hints that you need your home back. Ask them what their plans are and don't make life too easy for them, as it isn't helping them at all in the long term. Be honest that you need time and space now to be your own woman. They'll have to understand.*

Q **My husband comes home late because he travels all over the state with his work. As I am back home before him, the routine has been for me to cook. But now that I'm menopausal I want to break free. What can I do?**

A *Your husband might enjoy coming home and putting on the apron. Can he cook a couple of times a week? You do a couple and leave the other days to be a spontaneous break from the routine as well. It doesn't matter who comes home first—it's the routine that needs fixing. You'll both enjoy a change of pace.*

42

Beautiful breasts

Your breasts will be different now from the ones you had before menopause began—they will be softer, smoother, and will probably have lost some of their fullness.

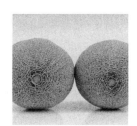

It doesn't mean they're not beautiful.

Beautiful breasts are in part a gift of nature, but are also in part the result of the care you take to protect and nourish them. Most of us no longer own the perky breasts we used to have when we were younger and this is partly because our bodies have stopped producing estrogen in the same quantity as before menopause started. Estrogen is the hormone that affects all the tissues in your body, including the breast tissue. When the level of estrogen begins to diminish, the texture and shape of the breasts begins to change.

This accounts for your breasts now being smaller in size and fullness. They will also begin to sag during menopause because of the partial deterioration of glandular tissue that had previously protected the firmness of your breasts. Most of the connective tissue in your breast is composed of a fibrous protein called collagen that needs estrogen to keep it healthy. Without estrogen your breasts lose their elasticity and change shape. Your nipples could also become less pronounced, although this varies from woman to woman.

Here's an idea for you... **Checking your breasts regularly for any lumps, soreness, or discharge is a must when you are menopausal. You should also have your breasts screened every two years once you reach the age of 50.**

The breast is also composed of fat and the pectoral muscle gives the breast its support, but no exercise will ever dramatically alter the structure or shape of your breasts—although a well-toned body will hold a pair of breasts better and make them appear firmer. It is the firmness women seem to miss, and although I would never try cosmetic surgery on my breasts, it certainly works for many menopausal women. I still prefer trying out natural ways of working with my body, but if your breasts are really drooping then cosmetic surgery might be just the ticket for you.

There isn't a great deal you can do once menopause starts but there are a few things you can do to prevent further deterioration of breast tissue.

KEEP A STABLE WEIGHT

As your weight fluctuates, so does the size of your breasts. You've probably noticed that whenever you've been on a weight-reducing diet your breasts have been the first to lose fat—possibly the last place you wanted it to disappear from. But through menopause dramatic weight change is an enemy to your breasts. Your breasts will always lose volume if you lose fat, but they will lose even more fullness if you lose weight too fast. Through menopause it is very tempting to want to lose weight quickly and get back into some sort of shape. But never crash diet when you are menopausal; try to maintain a stable weight through eating sensibly as this really will protect your breasts. Once they have lost their substance it is almost impossible to get it back again.

See IDEA 25, *"Wow! You look great!,"* for more ways of making the most of your body and looking good.

Try another idea...

TRY TO SLEEP ON YOUR BACK

This way you do not put too much weight on your breasts; it might also help if your breasts are sore or sensitive now that you're menopausal.

TRY SLEEPING WITH A BRA ON

French women are said to sleep with their bras on; the one I asked said she does and that her mother also had a night bra. This bra is softer than a daytime bra and is to support the breasts while sleeping, and especially through menopause. You could try one of those soft bras with no hooks and eyes to irritate you while you sleep. They are easily available.

"I have only got little feet because nothing grows in the shade."

DOLLY PARTON

Defining idea...

POSTURE

The other thing you must do is take care with posture to help you feel confident about the body you are growing into throughout menopause. Your body is changing shape generally and your breasts are simply part of that change. Correct posture will help.

WHAT ELSE CAN I TRY?

Well, the latest craze from Asia is the use of acupuncture for breast augmentation. There are no scars, no unsightly consequences of surgery, but the end result offers no guarantee of any increase or improvement in breast composition. The session lasts about two hours so could be done during an extended lunch break. It doesn't work miracles and promises only to increase the volume of breast tissue through stimulating what is already there—so if there's not much left now that you are menopausal, the chances are that you'll still be left with your A cup.

Q   **I am 50 and menopausal, and not suffering too badly apart from my breasts, which feel so tender. I don't have any lumps and I was told to take evening primrose oil. Will this help?**

How did it go?

A   *Evening primrose oil capsules are easily available and should ease the pain you are experiencing. Try taking 40 milligrams of vitamin B_6 daily as well. As the skin on your nipples is thinner than that on most other areas of your body, make sure you wear loose clothing, since any tightness will make them feel worse.*

Q   **I dislike wearing bras but feel that now that I am menopausal I really should. Am I right?**

A   *If you still have firm breasts then wear a bra when you run or exercise. There are mixed opinions on the bra issue; maybe if you feel you need one now and then for extra support you could buy a pretty, soft cotton one to wear through the day.*

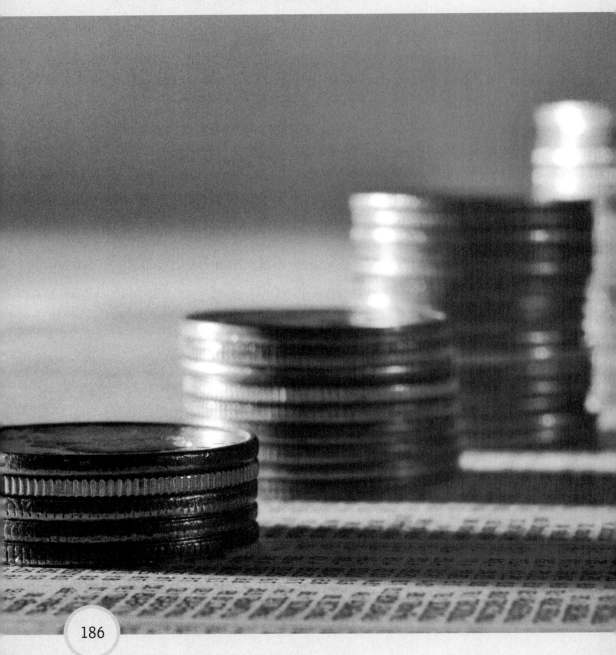

43

Money makes the world go round...

Menopause is a time in your life when you want freedom—and that means financial freedom, too.

If you have always shared a bank account then this might be a good time to set up your own checking or savings account.

Many couples share a bank account, which might have been useful when there were kids around or when one of you was employed and earning more than the other. A joint account means that all the hassle of bills can be managed easily and it's useful in that respect. But menopause is the right time to create new opportunities for yourself and also to allow yourself the chance to earn, save, and spend your own money. Having your own spending power is dignifying and liberating.

Even if you already have a separate account, or perhaps are single, read on as you may need to redefine your relationship with money anyway.

Lack of funds is one of the chief stressors in our society and creates more disharmony in our lives than almost anything else. When you are in menopause you want to limit opportunities for stress and learn to get your relationship with money

Here's an idea for you... **Once you have saved a little money, spend some wisely. Some suggestions:**
Travel: **Now is a great time to see the world. With the better part of your child-rearing days behind you, you can explore the world at your own pace and in just the way you would like to.**
Further education: **Signing up for a course at a college or your local community center can be liberating and fulfilling. You may even discover a new passion.**
Career: **Menopause is a great time to explore the world of work for your own benefits. You might even consider starting your own business.**

right. It doesn't mean you have to have tons of the stuff, but just make sure the money you do have you enjoy and feel is really "yours." Menopause is a good time to start saving—no matter how small the amount—to make you feel in control. Any kids will have have left home, so there might be a bit more for you.

But isn't it hard to keep it for yourself? As soon as you have some spare money, do you want to spend it on grandchildren or on another member of the family? Before you know it, the pot is empty again. Not that I'm saying don't treat others or help them out when you can, but know your boundaries and don't be afraid to say *no* to those who come knocking for money.

So how do you improve your relationship with money?

- Examine the relationship you already have with your money. Do you actually like it? You might find your fear of lack of it has created a love/hate relationship with it.

- Make a list of what you own and what you owe—include everything here from credit cards, overdrafts, loans, the lot. This part can be scary as most of us owe more than we own, and during menopause that's the last thing we want.

Look at IDEA 19, *All change*, to explore new ways of making changes.

Try another idea...

- Set an attainable savings plan. Even if you only save a small sum each month it's a start and will honestly kick in the "I am in control" factor. Many money experts agree that we invest too much emotion in our money and so never feel on a level footing with it and this damages our ability to save. Saving is only a way of thinking. Give it a try.
- Does money burn a hole in your pocket? Now that you are menopausal you mustn't let it. Leave your credit cards at home and use them only in emergencies.
- Do you envy other people—menopausal like you—who have lots of money? Well, that's negative thinking again and won't help you save. If you envy them you are, in effect, saying that you'll never have your own.
- The experts agree that everyone ought to give to charity on a regular basis as this keeps the "money flow" circulating in our lives.

If I ask you how much money you might need to make you happy, chances are you couldn't come up with a figure. In reality money and happiness aren't necessarily bedfellows, but money can make you feel more secure and in control, and gives you more choices about what to do in your life, something highly desirable during menopause.

Money and worry go hand in hand and it's time to break the grip money has over you. Let it come to you in menopause through changing your attitude toward it. Shopping is

"Money can't buy you happiness but it does bring you a pleasant form of misery."

SPIKE MILLIGAN

Defining idea...

such fun, but never really satisfies, does it? You buy something today and you want to shop again tomorrow. Only shop when you really want something and ignore all those impulse buys. Change your shopping activity and do something else to take its place. We waste so much in this society and you don't want to waste anything—ever.

How did it go?

Q **I am 46, in menopause, and want to know that the future looks bright. Should I be thinking about retirement savings yet?**

A   *All the experts would say you should and I agree—but don't forget to make sure you live each day not worrying about the future, but being careful and loving with your money today.*

Q **Since menopause I have managed to save regularly and would like to give something to my family for when they are older. So should I invest in savings bonds for my grandchildren so they have a nest egg later?**

A   *That's a lovely idea because your grandchildren will learn the value of money as they see it accumulate, and although you may not be around to see them spend it, you'll know you've provided them with something valuable.*

44

Get a little shut-eye...

Insomnia and interrupted sleep patterns are especially common during menopause, affecting over a third of all menopausal women.

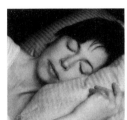

It's true that you need less sleep as you get older, but there is a difference between needing less sleep and having trouble sleeping when you're tired.

If you aren't waking up refreshed in the morning, do something about your sleeplessness. You're harming your health if you don't.

During the course of menopause, your ovaries gradually decrease production of estrogen and progesterone, a sleep-promoting hormone. The shifting ratios of hormones can be an unsettling process, sometimes contributing to the inability to fall asleep.

Is yours a general menopausal sleeplessness? Your mind is whirring, you wake up at 3:00 a.m. and look at the clock—then can't go back to sleep until dawn... Sleeping problems like difficulty falling asleep, trouble staying asleep, and restless sleep are common in menopause. Insomnia, in fact, is a common symptom of hormonal imbalance. Insomnia and related sleeping problems may have many causes, but the usual menopausal suspects are:

- Night sweats. These are produced by a surge of adrenaline that wakes your brain from sleep. Unfortunately, it may take time for your adrenaline to recede and let you settle down into sleep again.
- High stress levels. Being stressed causes adrenal malfunction and this can suppress levels of DHEA, a vital regulator of sleep. This is one way you might be paying for a hectic lifestyle.
- Alcohol or caffeine taken just before bedtime, which can often result in sleeplessness.
- Conflicts, worries, or problems that create anxiety that you have avoided dealing with or haven't been able to resolve happily.

Here's an idea for you...

Take a *cold* hot water bottle to bed with you if you are suffering from hot sweats, or even go one step further and take an ice pack to bed. Wrap it in a towel or two, make sure it doesn't leak, and it will cool down an overheating body and allow you to get some valuable shut-eye. It sounds dreadful but it really can work.

WHAT TO DO ABOUT IT

It's very important to avoid dependence on sleeping pills as a cure for insomnia. They may be needed to support you in the short term, but they create new problems without fixing the ones you already have. You could well find, like many menopausal women, that using natural things to help you sleep will be beneficial in the long term; they don't create a dependency. Herbs such as valerian and chamomile are good to take as teas last thing at night as they are naturally calming.

You might be magnesium deficient—the RDA for magnesium intake is 300 milligrams and it is good for your menopausal symptoms as it can ease your mood swings and fluctuations in memory. Magnesium is abundant in kelp, cashews, and pumpkin seeds.

Look at IDEA 13, *"Er, what was I saying?,"* to help you come to grips with other stresses that might be worrying you and therefore keeping you awake.

Try another idea...

I find that a few relaxation exercises help me unwind before bedtime and now that I do them regularly they trigger a natural feeling of being tired. I think the regularity has been really important for me. When you are under stress, your muscles tense and your breathing becomes shallow and rapid. One of the simplest ways to stop this stress response is to breathe deeply and slowly. Take time to practice this simple deep breathing each evening:

- Begin by breathing through your nostrils. Inhale for five counts, silently saying the word "in." Concentrate on breathing deeply. Fill your lower abdomen with air.
- To the count of five, exhale slowly, silently saying the word "out" as you let the air escape through pursed lips.
- Repeat this exercise for about two minutes. Gradually you will be able to build up to ten counts or higher. Increase your relaxation by imagining a peaceful scene or breathing in fresh air or pleasant smells.

You will always feel better if you sleep with a window open to let fresh air circulate. If it is safe to do so, keep it open all night, no matter what the weather. Be consistent with the times you go to bed and wake up. Build a very tight sleep structure by paying attention

"In a dark time, the eye begins to see."
THEODORE ROETHKE

Defining idea...

to your sleep environment. Turn off central heating at night whether you get the hot sweats or not, as a stuffy bedroom is not conducive to a good night's sleep and can make you feel drowsy instead of refreshed when you wake up. Change your bed linens often and always go for cotton so your body can breathe.

I wish you a good night!

Q **I just found a sleep routine and suddenly my husband has decided this is a good time to start snoring. I am at my wit's end. I really need my sleep after being deprived for so long. What can you recommend?**

A *Have you tried rolling him back onto his side again? If you put a pillow between you it can stop him from rolling onto his back. He may also need to reduce his weight as this might be making him snore. There are all sorts of remedies and cures for snoring and your pharmacist can offer you advice.*

Q **I always used to have a nightcap before going to bed; it was a little ritual I enjoyed. I'm not sleeping too well now that I'm menopausal, though. Should I stop my nightcap?**

A *A little alcohol seems to be beneficial in that it helps to improve digestion and is a relaxant as well. But much more than a glass or two of wine a day can create sleep problems—it blocks REM dreaming and can cause insomnia. Try limiting drinking alcohol with your evening meal and replace your alcoholic nightcap with a cup of warm soy milk sweetened with honey.*

45

Are you thinking what I'm thinking?

Now that you are menopausal, do you find yourself thinking far more than you used to?

The most precious resource we have is our time. Our lives are the sum total of what we do with that time. Isn't it worth spending even more of it thinking?

No, not simply reshuffling existing thoughts and ideas, but really trying to grapple with ideas, philosophies, and trying to make sense of the world you inhabit. You no longer need to be entertained every spare moment you have and, in fact, you'll probably be hitting the "off" button on the television far more during menopause. So why not replace that TV time with thinking? Now that you're menopausal it will be so rewarding if you can take time to think—and know that thinking will bring you closer to who you are and why you do the things you do. Many of the problems and challenges of our lives are not easy and they're not simple. They require thoughtful consideration.

WHAT TO DO

Take a "thinking" break when you allow yourself time to do nothing else but think. Thinking will boost your energy bank and give you the chance to see the bigger picture of your life, for yourself. Here's some help.

HOW TO BEGIN

- It doesn't matter where you are as long as you can close your eyes for a few minutes.
- Try not to be disturbed by anyone, and have a notebook ready for when the process is over so you can record everything of importance in your thinking time.
- Then take a few deep breaths and think of the subject you need clarification on…

GETTING ON WITH IT

You could be thinking about your own menopause and all the things that are happening to you right now. It could be about your relationship, your career, your home, or anything that's on your mind but stuck in the background for much of your time. The trouble with these background thoughts is that they can influence how we behave without our being aware of it. So you might dread looking for a new job, but deep down you know it's what you really want. If you don't think beyond the dread then the worry keeps you unhappy or bored at work and in turn that can make you feel ill—as it robs you of the feel-good factor and produces stress. Through

Here's an idea for you…

Menopause is not the beginning of mental decline. Instead, it is a time to expand your knowledge and embrace new ideas. Reflect on your past and acknowledge your emotions. Read books, magazines, and newspapers to absorb new ideas.

menopause, when it is vital to maintain good health and a positive spirit, it is time to deal with these "wallpaper worries" and think them through. It takes time and patience but the payoff is a life you feel more in control of.

IDEA 51, *Am I going crazy?*, will help you explore other ways of working with your mind and your imagination through menopause.

Try another idea...

Take one clear topic at a time and bring it to the front of your mind. Ask yourself a question about this issue and ask it again so you are clear on what you want to think about.

Now sit back and let the thinking process begin. Simply allow this deeper part of you to tell you the way forward through images, words, and ideas. Don't stop when you think you have the answer but ask the question again and insist on staying with it in your mind.

When you are ready, open your eyes and for a few minutes go over what has just happened. Write down every feeling, thought, and image you had while you were in free-fall thinking, and later put it together to see what you are being told to do.

You will have a sense of what the right thing is for you to do. Clarity is power. And clarity comes from thinking. It sounds so easy but at first it takes time to allow thoughts in—you might find yourself trying to contradict what you are thinking and this can be irritating to begin with.

There is an art to thinking and the best way to think productively is to do it regularly. If you want to change something in your life, set aside precious thinking time. Now that you are in menopause you want to experience the freedom that thinking brings about, and productive thinking really can affect your health for the better.

"Thinking is the hardest work there is, which is probably the reason so few engage in it."
HENRY FORD

Defining idea...

197

How did it go?

Q   **I have the best intention of changing my life, but now that I am menopausal all I want to do is relax and watch TV when I get home from work. I feel my life is a constant battle between what I actually do and what I know I should be doing. Will this thinking suit me?**

A   *At some point, you have to commit to the changes you want to make. Don't limit yourself to thinking the changes have to be made while you are at home, after a day's work. Instead, begin to make the changes while you are at work, through thinking about what needs to be done. Then you are halfway there.*

Q   **I find it so hard to let go and do the thinking exercises or even to try out meditation. My mind buzzes and whirrs all of the time. Would a course in hypnotherapy help me unwind enough to try thinking clearly?**

A   *Hypnosis is one way you can achieve that state between being awake and being asleep. Maybe you could ask yourself why you don't trust yourself enough to submit to your own thoughts. Is it a fear of losing control? If you stick with it, though, you will discover things about yourself and eventually you will find that being relaxed becomes easier. You will be able to learn how to do it yourself and begin to meditate or try free thinking.*

46

Excuse me, can you see me?

Your self-esteem is formed by your sense of self in the world and how you exist in it, and how you get along with the people in your life.

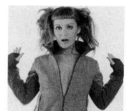

We don't get anywhere unless we have abundant levels of self-esteem. We need it to promote ourselves in the world "out there."

Low self-esteem when you are menopausal can be doubly difficult because you might not feel "visible" anymore as it is. Then there are always those days when you feel fat, boring, silly, and old, and you don't actually want to be seen anyway. Doesn't do much for your self-esteem, does it? When you're menopausal you need a strategy to get you moving out of a low-esteem day and straight into a better, more positive mode.

Your family might all be doing well in their relationships and professions or education, but you can't live your sense of self-worth through them. You have to find ways to achieve what you need to give you a sense of independence and success, and the knowledge that you can create the life you want to have.

Here's an idea for you... **Write yourself a long letter as though you were your own best friend and in it describe everything that you have done that you are proud of, and all the things you think you would tell yourself that you can still do. Highlight your strengths and point out all the times you have dealt with challenges in a noble and honorable way. Write this letter straight from your heart and keep it somewhere you can read it every day when you feel you are hitting a low ebb.**

To measure your self-esteem ask yourself what you would do in the following situation: You go and have your hair done by a top stylist, so it's costing quite a lot. You expect to look fabulous by the time they've finished with you. When they rinse the water out, the color is all wrong, you realize they haven't listened to you and they blow-dry it in the wrong way as well. You can't wait to get home to brush it all out so you look normal again.

If you have low self-esteem the chances are you pay for your terrible hairdo, thanking the hairdresser and even making a new appointment for a month's time. Low self-esteem means you wouldn't dream of asking them to redo it. Heightened self-esteem *insists* they redo it—and that they cover the cost.

HOW TO REPROGRAM YOUR LEVELS OF SELF-ESTEEM

- Ignore what anyone else says or thinks about you. This one takes practice, but stick with it and repeat to yourself that it's irrelevant whether they like you or don't like you. You are not here for everyone's approval.
- Take one step at a time and carefully "clock" events you know have knocked down your confidence. Retrace the moment and notice where you could have altered the course of events. Make a note of that.

Increasing levels of self-esteem at home means:

■ Breaking habits so you don't feel guilty if the meal isn't on the table by 6:30 p.m. When life is too predictable it becomes dull; you have too much time to reflect on the negative and not the positive things that could be going on around you.
■ Experimenting with your clothes and décor. Your surroundings have such an effect on how you feel. Have a corner or room where you can be free to create your own sacred, private, and safe space.
■ Going out to eat midweek or seeing some friends spontaneously.
■ Going to the movies on your own. If you hate it you can always come home again before the end of the film.
■ Refusing to watch television for a whole week.
■ Reading about women and their lives—how they dealt with their career, relationship, and money issues.

Shake everything up and you can release a new vitality into your life and make a supreme effort to see off all your feelings of low self-esteem. Menopause is exactly when feelings like that are the very last thing you want, need, or have to live with—so ditch them.

Browse through IDEA 47, *What? You don't want to grow old?*, to discover ways to keep feeling strong about the future.

Try another idea...

"To learn new habits is everything, for it is to reach the substance of life. Life is but a tissue of habits."

HENRI FREDERIC AMIEL, diarist, poet, and philosopher

Defining idea...

How did
it go?

Q **I feel so down and hate my image now. I want to try to change my life but have a fear of trying anything new—and that includes new makeup, clothes, or hair as I am worried people at work will laugh at me or wonder what on earth I am doing. Any tips?**

A *You know exactly the response everyone would give you to this predicament: forget what anyone else thinks. But that is probably easier to say than to do. Could you change your appearance in stages, and not shock anyone and everyone by doing it all at once? You won't feel so self-conscious if you take it slowly and carefully and you would have time to adapt to your new self as well. Plus, by taking it slowly you are less likely to make mistakes—which would only defeat the purpose, wouldn't it?*

Q **I don't want to become aggressive every time someone doesn't "see" me. Is there another way of making my presence felt?**

A *There is no need to be aggressive at all but just be firm and stick to your guns. Imagine how a woman you really admire for her sense of self-worth might deal with a tricky situation and do the same. It might feel odd to begin with but you'll soon get the hang of it.*

47

What? You don't want to grow old?

Menopause is definitely a time when we think about our own mortality.

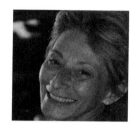

Possibly some of you have been secretly adding up how many years you might have left...

When my husband was given a new shovel recently he chuckled, saying that the shovel had a twenty-five-year guarantee with it—which was more than he had. That was a funny thought: that the shovel could be around when we were both gone.

Menopause can sometimes make us dwell on morbid events that we don't really want to think about. Yet menopause itself is certainly something to do with a kind of death—because it is the end of a way of life and a step in a different direction. Yet, did you know that menopause is a recent phenomenon in the history of mankind? In the past many women died before they reached the age of menopause.

203

Here's an idea for you...

If you have a fear of death then enjoying the simple things in life again might be beneficial. You could participate in daily walking through the park, make your own bread—anything that is grounding and definitely very earthy. If you keep your life simple the day seems longer and you become more in tune with the hours of the day and night again.

Death is probably the last taboo in our society, in the same way that menopause was not so long ago. In the past, certainly in your parents' experience, menopause would have been seen as a cruel punch line to your life. When it was talked about—if at all—it was in tones of fear and loathing. Menopause, the transition that marks the end of a woman's reproductive cycle, has attracted a host of negative feelings and superstitions, and many of these are hard to shake off.

Today you will work hard to get on with life throughout menopause and take it in stride. You'll discover a host of other women out there who really appreciate you, support you, and share their time and energy with you. I don't think I have ever valued people as much as now, since I've hit menopause.

What I want us to be sure of, though, is that although our life's work is nowhere near done, we are experiencing a mini-death and the surprise is that it has been better than we thought. Menopause, instead of closing us down, actually opens us up. A recent Gallup poll has said that women don't dread menopause as much as they once did, and the majority of women asked even said they were actually looking forward to it.

Defining idea...

"Death and taxes and childbirth! There's never any convenient time for any of them."

MARGARET MITCHELL, author

We talk about sex and menopause as though they were as mundane as a shopping list, but we feel safe with sex and menopause now. Maybe the time has come to feel safe talking about death? Maybe now that you are menopausal you could open up the topic of death a little so we can become a society without fear of death. We are a society obsessed with films and dramas about murders and could witness horrible, violent deaths almost daily if we wanted to, and yet most of us are afraid of it.

See IDEA 17, *Now you've found religion*, for other ways to find peace of mind and inner security.

Try another idea...

We could all start by making our own small but valuable preparations for death by being ready—having a will made out, and including in it a note of where we would like to be buried or have our ashes scattered. This will renew our belief in the cycle of life and death and help us and those we love accept the death part more easily.

Once you free yourself from the burden of the fear of death and face it, the fear goes. If you make your peace with death and do all in your power to have everything in place, and lead a healthy, creative lifestyle, then you can continue with your life secure in the knowledge that you have done and are doing all you can to make life better for not only yourself but those you love as well.

"If you were going to die soon and had only one phone call to make, who would you call and what would you say? And why are you waiting?"

STEPHEN LEVINE, poet

Defining idea...

205

How did
it go?

Q   I don't think I am a morbid person but I have been dreaming
     about death and dying so much since I started menopause that
     I am beginning to wonder if there is something wrong with me.
     I am always the one who is dying. Do you think my dreams are
     trying to tell me something?

A   *Yes, they most definitely are but I don't think it's so much about death as
     about new life. According to Rabbi Yehuda Berg, in* Kabbalah: The Dreams
     Book, *when you dream that you are the one who passes away, then this
     symbolizes a longer life for you.*

Q   My mom died when I was just a kid and I feel so sorry that she
     never saw my children or grandchildren. I keep looking at photos
     of her and it makes me very sad. I desperately want to believe in
     life after death but just can't. How can I keep her memory with-
     out a religion?

A   *Many women turn to spiritual things when they are menopausal since it
     seems to offer them a focus and clarity about the meaning of life. What
     happened to you is cruel but you can consider the ways your children have
     inherited some of your mother's characteristics and see life as a continuum.
     Then she is always with you, in a way.*

48

Sticky moments

Sometimes being stuck in a rut at work, in a bad relationship, with a financial matter, or with a dull social life can seem insurmountable.

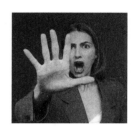

The trick is to change your approach to whatever has kept you stuck.

During menopause, you will want new challenges and more options. There's nothing as bad as feeling you can't move forward, and that every time you try you just end up where you started. Stuck!

If you deal with an issue in the same old way and live off hope, then all you get is more of the same, and the more frantic the hope becomes. You have to be proactive in those areas of your life you feel discontented about and make an active decision to change. Menopause is change incarnate and the old ways of dealing with most of your life are now outmoded and need a revamp.

With your career or job, it is exactly right to make yourself believe that *now* is the perfect moment to ask for a career change, promotion, sideways shift. Now is perfect to retrain, reconsider, and not feel like an automaton waiting to retire before the fun can begin again. It's probably best to think of life as a continuum where retirement doesn't actually ever happen.

Here's an idea for you... **The best way to get over feeling stuck is to get moving. Walk everywhere: take the stairs instead of the elevator, jump up and down a few times a day to defy gravity. As you move let your hands and arms flop, make silly noises—anything to get you away from who you think you are. Tai chi is good for physical and mental toning as it improves balance, flexibility, and, after a while through regular practice, you will be able to recognize the first symptoms of being stuck as they come along and then work to eliminate them before they get ahold on you.**

Imagine yourself in the best job ever, doing what challenges, inspires, and connects you to the source of your happiness. Why would you ever want to leave that and retire? If your job is not satisfying then, believe me, now is the time to learn, study, get out there and change things.

Being stuck in a bad relationship is different to being in one in need of a makeover. Take responsibility and don't blame your other half for all your ills. Blame makes you a victim. Stand before yourself and write a list—a totally honest and frank list—of everything you have done to create the relationship you are now stuck in. Is there a light somewhere you can follow to make the relationship work again? Do the right thing: Check with yourself and see where you can make changes. As soon as you begin to make those changes the rest follows. Try to see it as an adventure, not something to be gloomy about. Menopause is an excellent opportunity to create all the swift changes you would like to see happen in your life. Use your newfound intuition to assist you along the way. But do something, even if it is telling your partner you love him or her and that you want this relationship to work out.

There is a wonderful therapy called "the metamorphic technique" that isn't too well known, but people who have used it really love it. I am a convert and think it works wonders. The therapy works on the principle that we are all born with a memory of pre-birth events and especially about the time we were conceived. The therapist works to release the memories and all the patterns of behavior that come with it. I had a session and was asked to sit in front of the therapist, a truly lovely woman, while she gently massaged the inner sides of my feet from the heel to the toe. Then she took my hands and worked from my thumb to my wrist before working on my head. She chatted while she worked; the therapy isn't at all "precious" but remarkably relaxing. She says that by moving the "memory" we are enabled to move on and get out of situations where we find ourselves stuck. Why not search online for a therapist near you?

Anything at all you are feeling stuck about can be removed if you come at it from a different perspective. Don't wait until tomorrow.

While you are making changes in how you live you might want to make sure you are looking after your body at the same time. See IDEA 6, *Give yourself a good going-over*, for ways of keeping yourself in mint condition.

Try another idea...

"We do not see things as they are but as we are."
JEWISH PROVERB

Defining idea...

How did it go?

Q **I am a creature of habit but while I have been menopausal I have noticed subtle changes taking place in my mind about what I would like my relationship to be like. I would like to let my partner have more of a say in how we do things but I have always had the upper hand. How can I let go?**

A *Tell him exactly what the problem is and ask him to tell you what you can do together to make the relationship more equal. If he can find a way to work with you—through both of you talking about everything before any decisions are made—he will get the hang of it. You will respect him more and find more freedom through sharing, not less.*

Q **When menopause started I thought my life was over but now I find I want to travel and explore the world alone. Am I being foolish?**

A *There are plenty of safe ways to travel. Go somewhere you already know by yourself to begin with, so you have a bit of a net and can feel what it's like to do things alone. Then, if you found it comfortable, you can move to new destinations. You know all the safety rules and if you stick to them you should have the travels of a lifetime. Enjoy.*

49

OK, but make it a small one

Headaches? Depression? Hangover? Can't hold your liquor anymore?

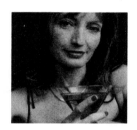

Isn't it annoying how, not very long ago, you could have a little G and T, or a glass of wine, at any time of the day and it slipped down very easily?

These days you probably need to eke out your allowance with such care and precision it hardly seems worth the trouble of having a drink.

Drinking too much, as we all know now, is never good for anyone whatever their age. Drinking too much while going through menopause is a big mistake. Women are more sensitive to the impact alcohol has anyway, owing to their generally smaller physique and higher ratio of body fat. Alcohol also makes you pack on the weight, wrecks your bones, and does untold damage to your skin—so, in effect, it adds years to your face.

I really dislike those magazine articles that make it seem that if you drink alone you're a raving alcoholic. A few years ago when I moved temporarily to Amsterdam, I was alone and I loved my evening gin and tonic. Many of us drink alone

Here's an idea for you... **Organic wine has fewer chemicals and pesticides than non-organic, so it might be better to do yourself a favor and stick to that if you suffer from headaches. Organic wines are easier to find now and supermarkets will advise you as to which wines are organic—or even vegan—if you ask. Experiment to find out what you can safely drink without feeling grim the following morning.**

now and then and there's nothing nicer than having the house to yourself and enjoying a little cocktail. In fact, I think I drink less when I drink alone than I do when I am with friends.

However, as soon as menopause hit, the gin crippled me. I felt as though a knife was lodged in my eye. Red wine made it ten times worse and yet a few days later I'd be ready to try drinking again, hoping one little glass wouldn't hurt. I was angry that a simple pleasure had been taken away from me. Not all my menopausal friends had to give up alcohol and I wanted to be like them. As soon as I realized the inflated importance I had put on my solo drink, it lost its value and I no longer needed it. That sounds very easy but it was a battle for a while. Far from seeing yourself as being a desperate lush, find out why and what you associate with that little drink you enjoy on your own.

If you are concerned you could have a booze issue, no matter how small, do something about it today. Don't put it off. Menopause gives you enough to think about without the added burden of alcohol coursing through your veins messing everything up. Alcohol never changes anything for the better—except in the very short term—and as you will have learned to your cost, the old feelings flood back the moment the booze hit is over.

Alcohol lowers your libido and as a sparkling sex life is more important than a bottle of fizz, see IDEA 10, *Am I still attractive?*, for ways to put the passion back on the agenda.

Try another idea…

The bottle of champagne in the fridge can wait until you've got something to celebrate, like the fact that you've cut down on alcohol. As soon as I stopped my three months of abstinence, I held a little champagne bash, had two glasses, and felt as high as a kite. It was lovely.

Try non-alcoholic cocktails, as they don't dehydrate but will cram you with vitamins and other goodies—and as they are quite intensive to prepare they certainly stop you from thinking about anything alcoholic at all. Make them as spectacular as you can; the color and the smells will give you a high and everyone loves them. Most restaurants offer a decent range of fruit-based cocktails, too.

"I feel sorry for people who don't drink. When they wake up in the morning, that's as good as they're going to feel all day."

FRANK SINATRA

Defining idea…

213

How did it go?

Q **I love a glass of wine and don't want to give it up altogether— just cut down. My friends seem to hate the idea and are doing everything in their power to prevent me from sticking to the one glass. What can I say to them?**

A *Can't friends be a pain sometimes? You try to do what is best and they try to sabotage your efforts. Let them know in advance that you won't be drinking that much and take your own non-alcoholic drink as well as a bottle of wine for them. If you absolutely insist that they don't buy you a round then they ought to realize you mean business. You don't have to be nasty, just firm. Put your hand over your glass or just don't drink any extra they add. When you can, let them know you need help and support while you are trying to cut down and that their attitude, while understandable, is not remotely helpful.*

Q **I think I'm becoming dependent on alcohol. I used to get by on a couple of glasses but now we can get through a couple of bottles of wine with our supper easily. My husband tells me not to have more than two glasses a day but once I start I can't seem to stop. How can I?**

A *As you are drinking more than a couple of glasses a day then your husband is quite right and it's time to put the brakes on your drinking. Can you change your eating time so you mess up the routine a little? Part of the problem could be that you are stuck in this routine and entrenched in a fixed way of doing things. If you can, stop altogether and give yourself a month off the booze. When you come back to it, your tolerance level will be lower and you will drink less.*

50

Gorgeous, sexy, and I hate you!

I still can't help a whiff of nostalgia as I see those gorgeous young women today dressed to kill, even in jeans and baggy sweaters, looking all healthy and glowing.

Don't think I really hate you...

It's just that some days I miss the way my face, like yours, never looked crumpled in the morning… I bet when you wake up your hair will do whatever you tell it to, and your feet aren't ablaze with blisters and corns from tottering around on ridiculously high heels like the ones I wore yesterday…

To add insult to injury, they even look so attractive in those aerobic classes. I used to huff and puff while trying to smile and look as though I was finding it so easy, but now I go speed walking instead—alone. I love being around younger women, just not when I am undressed. If you see yourself as little more than a withered old prune then comments such as, "You were probably gorgeous in your day" make you feel a million times worse. "This is still my day," I say.

Here's an idea for you...

Buy a close younger female friend something lovely she can keep forever—a piece of jewelry or a beautiful book. When it's her turn to become menopausal she can be reminded of you and that she knew you when you were menopausal. It will remind her that just as you got through in the best way possible, so can she.

But, thank goodness, we no longer see younger women as the enemy ready to whisk our men away from us. Men have grown up now and want us as the mature older women we are. Don't they?

Young women are great to have around and can inspire you with their energy. They're full of wacky, wonderful ideas and will remind you of your own more youthful years. Younger women are powerful and are generally fiercely loyal to their older female friends. A younger woman will experiment with her clothes, and this is a great way for you to pick up new tips as well as discover what's new on the market. They can also give you a sense of confidence about trying out anything new or any idea you might have, whether it's about your career, relationship, or even a vacation.

So cultivate friendships with them, flirt with them, get to know what makes them tick, and ask their advice; offer your own when it is asked for. Get them to advise you on your hair or makeup, as a young, fresh perspective might just be what you are looking for. They are a different generation and will have a different set of rules to live by.

In return, you, as the older and wiser woman, might be able to teach the younger women in your life some valuable life skills as well. Keep your advice positive and life-affirming. Younger woman have enough to be alarmed about: They might get fat, lose their looks, be dumped for an older woman twice their age, and have pregnancy and children to think about... You can teach them about their health, relationships, and about parenting.

Read IDEA 12, *What do you mean you "feel like a woman"?*, for more about women and how important they are.

Try another idea...

A little positive whispering about the benefits of menopause might be more than welcome, as well. Let younger women know that menopausal years aren't a signal that everything is over, just a sign that another stage has begun. Imagine if you had been repeatedly informed that menopause would be one of the most exhilarating experiences of your life and an event to be greeted with excitement and welcomed with open arms. Imagine how you would have felt. Might it even have changed the menopause you are now having?

You could inform the young women in your life that one of the ways you are reaping the benefits of being menopausal is by staying in touch with your intuitive self and that your life has been made richer as a result. Teach them how to use their own intuition, and how to trust it.

Spending all your time longing for your lost youth gives everyone the shivers—younger women will dread getting old and you will be wasting your time hankering after the impossible. So don't do it.

"Each friend represents a world in us, a world possibly not born until they arrive, and it is only by this meeting that a new world is born."

ANÄIS NIN

Defining idea...

How did it go?

Q **My partner went off with a younger woman some years ago just as I entered menopause and now I have met someone new but am terrified he will do the same. Can you help?**

A *While life offers no guarantees it is probably fairly safe to say he has chosen you, an older woman, later in life, so wants you and not someone younger. If you are through menopause, then you will be feeling more settled and ready to cope with any of life's challenges—so put the past behind you and enjoy the man who has chosen you as his lover.*

Q **A younger woman at work used to look up to me as her mentor but recently, after a drink with her, I told her too much about myself and now I have the sense that she has backed off. What can I do to restore the relationship?**

A *She has a lesson to learn, and so do you. If she was captivated by an illusion of you and not the real you then it is good for her to have seen the truth about you—that you are still the very same woman she admired so much. On the other hand, sometimes it is wise to stop before booze loosens the tongue too much. You could make light of it and tell her there are a million more skeletons in your closet...or ask her outright if she was shocked or offended by what you told her. It would be useful for you to know why she has had a change of heart.*

51

Am I going crazy?

I know it sounds funny but I think every menopausal woman knows exactly what I mean.

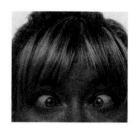

It's not that you are actually going round the bend, but you experience more days when you think you are.

The emotional roller coaster you might well find yourself on at the moment, producing all those feelings of irritability, mood swings, melancholy, and worry, is most likely brought on by the hormone changes you are experiencing. Decreased levels of estrogen can make you more vulnerable to stress, depression, and anxiety. This lack of estrogen also affects your REM sleep and when this is disrupted it can make you feel edgy, tired, and lethargic. Just when you feel you really need your sleep is exactly when it seems to evade you. Sometimes I had mood swings verging on sheer rage and terror—and these weren't helped by me endlessly wandering around the house between 3:00 and 5:00 a.m. like some demented Lady Macbeth, on the search for something but unsure what.

It's certainly a strange time and one that takes some getting used to. When you have a menopausal madness day it takes a huge effort to sift through the anxiety to spot the positive aspects of menopause. It also takes a big dose of trying to be

*Here's an
idea for
you...*

Try something brand new to match the new you. What about a bungee jump? Try something you would never normally have done in a million years. Not only will it amaze your friends, but you will have set yourself a personal goal to overcome a fear—and that's what menopause wants you to do. Overcoming fears is strengthening and liberating. Go for it right in the middle of menopause as it is utterly distracting and will help you with feelings of slight menopausal insanity.

objective and telling yourself that this is a learning curve and although things will never return to how they used to be, you will find an equilibrium and certainly feel better knowing time menopause is a time rich in self-discovery.

Menopause is probably pushing for you to experience a heightened midlife transition because it wants to find ways of moving you in a new and different direction. This is menopause telling you that midlife is a crucial time for you to sort out, clear out, and get out. It's the time for you to be heard and seen.

Sometimes you will think your madness is all your own doing and actually forget you are going through this huge transition. Here are some examples of what might be happening, and what you could do about it:

- You could find that the people you have always surrounded yourself with might no longer hold the same appeal, but on the other hand you could form even stronger attachments to some of them. What to do? Realize that you are the one changing so everything else in your world will appear different at the moment, won't it?

- You could be bored at home doing the same things day in and day out. What to do? Change the way you do things or even stop doing them for a while. See what happens if you no longer behave in your usual way.
- You might find you can't resolve issues with people as easily as you could, that you are taking things more seriously these days and yet you can see the funny side of a situation as well. What to do? Opt for laughing whenever you can. It's all too serious as it is and if you can see a spark of humor, go for it.

For ways to clear up the past and ease the way for the future, read IDEA 37, *Unresolved matters.*

Try another idea...

Don't dismiss your strange days too quickly, though, as there's so much you can learn through this stage and feeling slightly crazy has its compensations. It can propel you to make leaps forward, leaps into the void. It could start you on the road to a creative process, encouraging you to take up something you never realized you wanted to, like horse riding, circus skills—miming and clowning—or catering for dinner parties. Whatever you feel your madness is inspiring in you, do it and see how it goes. Don't spend too long thinking about it or the moment will pass and you'll feel normal again.

"You're only given a little spark of madness. You mustn't lose it."

ROBIN WILLIAMS

Defining idea...

221

How did it go?

Q **I feel very much like I did when I was going through puberty now that menopause has begun. I keep thinking there is something wrong with me and I'll feel normal again in a minute but of course I won't, will I?**

A *Once again, your hormones are ready to wreak havoc on your body, your emotions, and your mental faculties. This time around, however, you're a bit wiser, you have experience in dealing with change. You will find that what is happening to you will begin to feel normal very quickly, as long as you care for yourself and accept that menopause has begun. Don't fight menopause—work with it.*

Q **I cry at the drop of a hat and have this overwhelming desire to live in Mexico. I took myself there last year and think it would be the perfect place for me to spend the rest of my menopausal days. I can't help but feel I'm going nuts. Am I?**

A *Seeing the process as natural might help you stop thinking "there is something wrong with me" and help you realize that the feelings and changes associated with menopause are quite natural. In fact, they are experienced by most other menopausal women on the planet. If you take time to recognize the stages you are going through then this can help you make sense of what is otherwise a chaotic and confusing time in your life. Mexico sounds like fun. Could you spend six months there working or writing about your travels? I like that idea and can see the title already:* A Mexican Menopause.

52

How is it for you?

Many of the women I have spoken to about menopause gave me such huge insights that I think you ought to have some examples of what they've been saying...

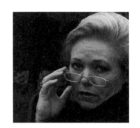

You all know women who are going through menopause and everyone has a different tale to tell. Here are some:

"I felt liberated as soon as my periods stopped. I used to have such bad period pains right up to the last one. They didn't fizzle out, though—I had one heavy one and that was it. I don't look back and wish I had those fertile years back at all. I'm hugely relieved my 'fertile' years are over."
—Ms. S., age 54

"I think I have spent a lot of my menopause running from mirror to mirror because I couldn't believe how much weight I had put on, and kept putting on. I think you have to take control of your weight as soon as you notice that first extra inch when you're menopausal because before you know it you're huge."
—Mrs. H., age 59

"I'm finding menopause the worst time of my life! I can't wait for it to be all over—and of course it's lasted five long years already. What do I recommend? A stiff whiskey every night, lots of chocolate cake, and a personal trainer."
—Mrs. M., age 50

"Nothing could have prepared me for the roller coaster of emotions I was going to feel right from day one of menopause. I could feel depressed and buoyant all at once some days. I don't think I would have liked to have gone through life without these feelings even though they were very unpredictable. I feel as though I was delving deep into who I was."
—Mrs. T., age 50

Here's an idea for you...

Begin a creative endeavor now that you are menopausal. Menopause brings with it so much energy that you might like to channel this into a project, large or small. You could learn to paint, draw, take fantastic photographs, write a book, or take up poetry. Do something to soak up the world around you—now that you are seeing it through menopausal eyes.

"I couldn't believe it when I realized menopause had started. I was 54 and even at my age I was in a sort of denial about it. I think I felt happier not knowing I was menopausal as I never knew what to expect and had heard so many negative things about menopause. In the end, though, I have to say it wasn't as bad as I had dreaded it might be—well, I'm still in it, I think. I do look after myself, though: Take lots of supplements and eat the right things."
—Ms. E., age 56

"I made the fridge my best friend: As soon as I feel a hot flash coming on I grab a bag of frozen vegetables and pop it on my head. Instant relief."
—Mrs. B., age 48

See IDEA 8, *Moving mountains*, to keep you running right to the end of the road.

Try another idea…

"I couldn't even look at a bottle of red wine as soon as menopause started—I would get such a headache. I was so angry. I looked the same but couldn't do the same things anymore. I tried white wine and that made no difference, I would be in bed with a raging headache within minutes of drinking. I miss my wine and hope it settles down soon."
—Mrs. Y., age 46

"Sex? I used to love sex, but my sexual desire was all over the place and intercourse felt different. It wasn't painful exactly but I certainly didn't want it to go on for hours. Just a few minutes was quite enough, which was a shame for my husband, as he'd been reading up about tantric sex and wanted to give me the time of my life and not ejaculate for hours on end. No thanks."
—Mrs. H., age 47

"Am I an old woman? I suppose I am but I don't feel it. I do feel different, yes, but older? Not really, no. I think the herbs I take and the acupuncture I have been doing help keep me

"I was very aware of a feeling of professional menopause. I felt that I needed new horizons for my own self as well as my work. And it was a wonderful challenge to take on a completely new theater of life and experience and try to fit it into fictional form."
JOHN LE CARRE

Defining idea…

in balance both physically and mentally. I think that women are probably at their most beautiful when they are menopausal, something about what they have been through and are going through really shows."

—Ms. W., age 58

How did it go?

Q   I haven't had the easiest menopause but I regret telling my daughters how bad it was when it might not be like that for them. I didn't do the things I now realize I could have done to make it a better experience. How can I put things right?

A   *It's never too late to tell them that you could have made it better. They'll be very pleased to hear that. Explain that part of the pain is your body sorting out all sorts of issues from the physical to the emotional and that it gets easier as they are cleared up. More than that, let them see you are still learning and growing and enjoying all the processes your body is going through.*

Q   I am so happy to be an older menopausal woman. Some of my friends think I am round the bend because I feel so different these days—so like the woman I was born to be. Can menopause really do that?

A   *You aren't the first to express that feeling and hopefully won't be the last. Women do return to a state of mind they recognize, as though they are being put back on course again and are given a second chance to follow their true nature. If you don't fight it, but trust your body and instincts during this time, it is a wonderful place to be.*

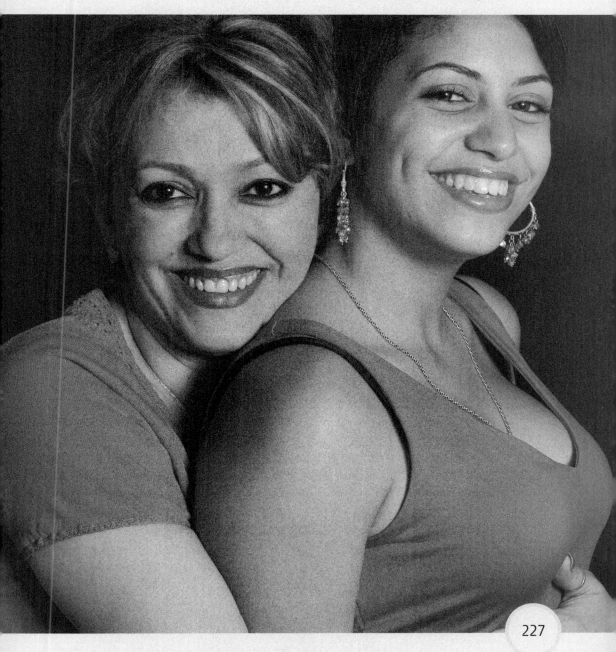

Where it's at...

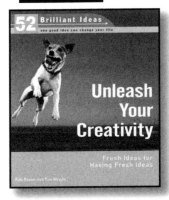

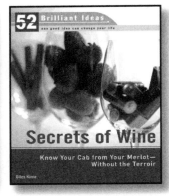

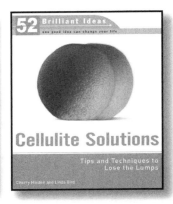

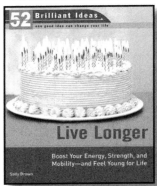

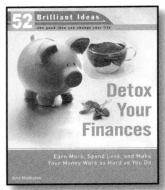

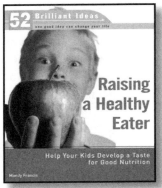

UNLEASH YOUR CREATIVITY
978-0-399-53325-9

LIVE LONGER
978-0-399-53302-0

SECRETS OF WINE
978-0-399-53348-8

DETOX YOUR FINANCES
978-0-399-53301-3

CELLULITE SOLUTIONS
978-0-399-53326-6

RAISING A HEALTHY EATER
978-0-399-53339-6

 An imprint of Penguin Group (USA)

T10A.0108

one good idea can change your life

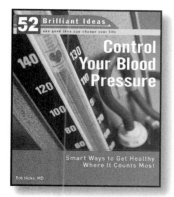
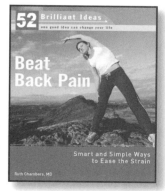
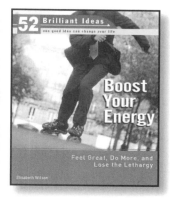

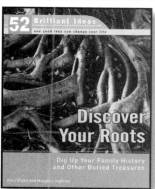
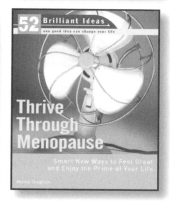
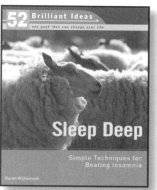

CONTROL YOUR BLOOD PRESSURE
978-0-399-53425-6

DISCOVER YOUR ROOTS
978-0-399-53322-8

BEAT BACK PAIN
978-0-399-53389-1

THRIVE THROUGH MENOPAUSE
978-0-399-53437-9

BOOST YOUR ENERGY
978-0-399-53432-4

SLEEP DEEP
978-0-399-53323-5

Available wherever books are sold or at penguin.com